StretchSmart

Dynamic stretching to improve
the way you feel and move

Adam Weiss, D.C.
Author of The BackSmart Fitness Plan

Library of Congress of Cataloging-in-Publication Data
Weiss, Adam, D.C.
StretchSmart: Dynamic stretching to improve the way you feel and move/ Adam Weiss
p.cm.
ISBN 978-0692576168
1. Stretching   2. Exercise   3. Injury prevention.   I. Title

Interior photos by Wesley Park
Cover design by Susan Weiss
This book is for educational purposes. It is not intended as a substitute for individual fitness, health, and medical advice. Please consult a qualified health care professional for individual health and medical advice. The information given is designed to help you make informed decisions about your body and health. The suggestions for specific foods, nutritional supplements, and exercises in this program are not intended to replace appropriate or necessary medical care. Before starting any exercise program, always see your physician. If you have specific medical symptoms, consult your physician immediately. If any recommendations given in this program contradict your physician's advice.. Be sure to consult your doctor before proceeding. Mention of specific products, companies, organization or authorities in this book does not imply endorsement by the author or the publisher, nor does mention of specific companies, organizations, or authorities in this book imply that they endorse the book. The author and the publisher disclaim any liability or loss, personal or otherwise, resulting from procedures in this program. Neither the author nor the publisher shall have any responsibility for any adverse effects arising directly or indirectly as a result on information provided in this book. Internet address and references given in this book were accurate at the time the book went to press. Product pictures, trademarks, and trademark brand names are used throughout this book to inform the reader about various proprietary products and trademarks and are not intended to copyright, or other rights nor imply any claim to mark other than that made by the owner. No endorsement of the information contained in this book has been given by owners of such products and trademarks, and no such endorsement is implied by inclusion of product pictures or trademarks in this book.

CONTENTS

ACKNOWLEDGMENTS   **v**

PROLOGUE   **vii**

INTRODUCTION   **viii**

CHAPTER 1
THE ULTIMATE STRETCHING PROGRAM FOR
MUSCLE TENSION RELIEF   **1**

CHAPTER 2
STIFF AS A BOARD? PROTOCOL FOR EASING INTO IT   **14**

CHAPTER 3
PERFECT POSTURE—BEYOND STRUCTURAL
LIMITATIONS AND IMPROVING HOW YOU LOOK   **24**

CHAPTER 4
WALL STRETCHES—A PARTNER
TO ENHANCE YOUR FLEXIBILITY   **42**

CHAPTER5
TOWEL STRETCHES—HEALING MOVES HOW
TO RELIEVE AND PREVENT STIFFNESS GENTLY   **57**

CHAPTER 6
CHAIR AND BALL STRETCHES:
RELEASE NERVOUS TENSION   **69**

CHAPTER 7
DYNAMIC MOVING STRETCHES   **91**

CHAPTER 8
SEQUENCE STRETCHES—WHEN YOU NEED TO
BYPASS A STICKING POINT IN YOUR FLEXIBILITY   **126**

CHAPTER 9
SUGGESTED STRETCHING ROUTINES FOR SPORTS   **133**

Dedicated to the memory of my father Michael Weiss
Who could make me smile and laugh at a drop of a hat! And still does.

ACKNOWLEDGMENTS

This book, like my past books, never would have seen the light of day if it weren't for the support and commitment of others. They include, first and foremost, my family. I am grateful to my mother. You are always there when I or someone else needs you! Amazing, and she still finds time to get her walk in too. Thanks goes to my dad, if I didn't have him in the back of my mind daily reminding me "Are you done with your book yet?" We both would laugh, I am working on it.

Much gratitude goes to my wife. She designs everything from the book cover, postcards, and website without clear direction from me but manages to produce something more exciting than I thought possible. For her humor, no matter how our day went we still manage to laugh before going to sleep.

My two children are what keeps me going. I offer them a special thank you for allowing me to explore every aspect of life with them, even if at times it may be over-sharing! In addition, I appreciate my son Brandon, for sharing his latest thoughts on a subject no matter how crazy the subject matter may be. Also, for trying to make me laugh daily. (Always smiling on the inside pal!). You are more and more like your grandfather every day and I thank you for that! Rachel, my sun shine! Your determination and pure will power never cease to amaze me! How I cherish our TV time, a book store, adventures, and making your lunch! Thank you for taking one for the team and eating at places where I can eat my chicken sandwich!

For my sister, the bravest person I know, when the world is falling apart around us your encouraging words "Think positive thoughts." reminds me that anything can be accomplished.

My brother thank you for taking me to see the Olympic athletes at the Pan Am games when I was a teenager. This is a memory I will never forget to this day the excitement and fun we had.

I am grateful to my photographer Wes, I learn something new each encounter during our twelve hour photo shoot and thank you for your detail in shooting this book. This book, like in the past, has been modeled by a friend who never says "no" when it comes to trying a new exercise or making it better after tweaking the movement, making it more challenging to her despair. A special thanks to you, Jackie.

I owe a debt of gratitude to my patients, who trusted me and my methods of care with each challenge they brought my way. I also thank the Pilates gang for allowing me to experiment with new exercises in class.

Finally thanks to you, my readers, for inspiring me to continue writing on the subject of exercise and for your supportive e-mails. From the first responders in London, to the Japanese flight attendant, Olympic athletes and hopefuls who have emailed me with questions from around the world, how we can improve upon ourselves through movement.

PROLOGUE

Why **read this book?** I know that I can make a difference and help you expand your flexibility; regardless of your age, how out of shape, or stiff you are, and however many past attempts you have made to commit to a flexibility routine. I have taught thousands of clients over the past 20 years. Improving your flexibility does not need to be as difficult as people make it out to be!

People often self-sabotage their own progress by placing mental barriers in their way towards getting fit. The human body has a memory pattern and thrives on being healthy and strong and more supple. I guarantee that when these exercises are incorporated into a daily routine, anyone attempting them will be able to increase his or her flexibility, improve muscle tone, shape, and posture. You will notice your overall health will be improved and you will be able to participate in your chosen physical activities. By combining these methods of exercise you can change your physical appearance by improving your posture—standing and sitting taller and in more relaxed positions, reducing joint and muscle tightness all while enhancing your flexibility.

INTRODUCTION

While there are books on the market today that have covered stretches from daily stretching to sport specific stretching, *StretchSmart* takes you instead through a series of dynamic functional stretching movements actively lengthening and relaxing major muscles groups while performing an easy to learn rhythmic series of exercises. *StretchSmart* will teach you how to eliminate improper straining and overcome structural limitations such as tight hamstrings, a stiff back, shoulder, or knees. *StretchSmart* will help you conquer "bad" chronic posture while preventing injuries at the same time.

StretchSmart will show a step-by-step method for improving your flexibility, even for those who think they were born "stiff," to provide a fuller range of motion in joints and muscles, for a more enjoyable lifestyle. It will improve your tennis or golf swing or just help you to bend over and tie your shoes.

StretchSmart will vastly enhance your body awareness and motion. There are no difficult positions to learn or get into and you will continue to benefit from these stretches. You will not have to hold awkward positions for a long period of time to improve your flexibility. While the *StretchSmart* exercises can be performed safely by all ages and fitness levels, simply following the instructions of gently moving the body through a series of movements using the path of least resistance will help you achieve a greater flexibility in a shorter period of time. These techniques have been used in providing therapeutic relief for thousands of my clients over the past 20 years at my center. And you can get the same positive results.

StretchSmart will offer a protocol for those who are "stiff as a board" to get on board to a healthy stretching routine, which they have been avoiding because of the difficulty in touching their toes or the discomfort associated with stretching for someone who has not done so in a very long time. *StretchSmart* will show you how to integrate stretching easily into your daily routine. Speaking of schedule, *StretchSmart* will appeal to those who are on the go and have only a few minutes a day to get in a workout, as well as the more athletic reader who wants to improve his or her range of motion to prevent injury.

CHAPTER 1

ULTIMATE STRETCHING PROGRAM FOR MUSCLE TENSION RELIEF

WHY YOU NEED TO STRETCH AND WHY IT DOESN'T HAVE TO HURT

By picking up this book you are one step closer to restoring your functional ability without the pain of getting there. By using exciting and challenging exercises, you'll increase your flexibility, which can help you in sports, training, and everyday life—from bending over and tying your shoes to better upright posture while standing and sitting. Stretching is a powerful part of any exercise program. Here's why—and how—to include stretching in your fitness routine.

THE KEY TO STRETCHING IS TO PREVENT INJURY

Whether you obtained your initial information from your sixth-grade gym teacher or picked up a few new moves at the gym, the key reason for stretching is to prevent injuries from occurring while doing other activities. Most people wait too late to start a stretching program, only seeking one after they have sustained an injury and need professional advice for their injuries. In most cases, they are given stretches to help them speed their recovery back to health.

In my center, most of my new patients have injured themselves by over-straining a stiff muscle group or joint, and these injuries could have been easily prevented by daily stretching. Not just a few minutes before an athletic event or workout but as a routine of awakening your body for the day ahead, during and at the end of your day to truly improve the way you move and feel.

TO IMPROVE RANGE OF MOTION

I was introduced to the importance of stretching early on in age when I joined a martial arts club that emphasized kicking. So we spent a lot of time stretching our legs, hips, and lower back muscles to improve our range of motion for better performance and power and speed in our kicks. Today, later in life, I find it is so important to stretch to move in and out of positions that I would never had thought about at a younger age.

Your goal is to improve your motion, period. If you want to excel at your chosen sport or just want to work out the kinks out in your body, you need to incorporate stretching. Most people go about it the wrong way so they disregard it completely, or make a half-hearted attempt at swinging their arms in big circles or twisting themselves side-to-side at the waistline for a few times.

So many former professional and amateur athletes' careers are cut short due to an injury that possibly could have been prevented if they had taken the time to improve their flexibility, not only their strength.

If you or someone you know "pulled" a muscle, was it a result of not thoroughly warming up and stretching from every angle possible?

Pulled, or micro tears in the muscle groups, can be prevented by stretching your muscles and allowing the fascia (thin but strong connective tissue) that surrounds the muscle to adapt to your new range of motion. This will give you more flexibility and prevent "pulled" muscles from occurring in the first place.

The *StretchSmart* technique of stretching will pinpoint individual muscle groups with compound movements to allow you to perform at your highest potential, rather than just isolate a single muscle. Thus it is a less painful way of stretching because you are using your muscles as a whole unit as they function in everyday activities.

These series of stretches will reduce your workload by removing tightness so you can move more freely throughout your entire body, not just in one area.

These *StretchSmart* stretches transport oxygen to your sore muscles and quickly remove toxins from your muscles so your recovery is faster from your other workouts, improving your overall flexibility.

BETTER FLEXIBILITY RESULTS IN LESS JOINT PAIN

Good flexibility is known to bring positive benefits to the muscles and joints by minimizing muscle soreness on a cellular level, while preventing future injury that might occur due to lack of motion, as well as improve efficiency in all your everyday activities and improve your quality of life and functional independence.

Rather than making your stretching attempts too brief, you'll be able to use *StretchSmart* routine to concentrate on your often neglected postural muscles that run throughout your entire body and have the tendency to be chronically stiff, in addition to stretching the major muscles groups in your body. By focusing on these muscles you'll utilize your time more efficiently and as your flexibility improves the movements become easier and more graceful.

StretchSmart is your comprehensive guide to the most important aspect of your fitness routine. Whether you're a weight lifter, tennis player, runner, golfer or a walker or simply trying to get the kinks out after a long day of sitting, Stretching Smart is a proven way to improve your sense of body movement and fitness. By lengthening your muscles and lubricating the joints, stretching smart will prevent injuries from occurring due to tightness. Stretching smart will also promote recovery and improve your posture and balance. Learning these series of stretches correctly will help you maximize your other workouts.

The following chapters of stretching movements are easy to use, and take you through every muscle group in the body with step-by-step instructions on these dynamic functional stretches. Most stretches can be done anywhere, at work, home or in the gym by using common household items such as a towel, chair and a wall to help you make stretching a fun and effective part of your daily routine.

Increasing flexibility can also improve quality of life and functional independence. Good flexibility aids in the elasticity of your muscles and provides a wider range of motion in the joints. It provides ease in the body movements and everyday activities. A simple daily task such as bending over and tying one's shoe is accomplished with better flexibility.

STRETCHING SHOULDN'T HURT

As you know by now, stretching offers an array of health benefits. But like any physical activity, it's not completely risk free. If you've been stretching for a while, you or someone you know has probably pulled a hamstring, or experienced some type of discomfort while stretching. Injuries can be great teachers. They invite you to uncover your stretching faults—misalignments or overzealous attempts to force your way into a position or to hold a position too long—and you learn to make corrections. But it's smart to learn the proper techniques, especially when it comes to your knee joints, hamstring tendons, sacroiliac joints, hip flexors and shoulder and neck regions. These parts are vulnerable to damage and take time to mend. With *StretchSmart* routine you'll learn ways to bypass the weak links that have been hindering your range of motion and you'll be able to improve upon your flexibility with a better understanding of how your body moves.

THE ROAD TO INJURY BY FORCING YOUR BODY INTO POSITIONS

Have you always found it difficult to touch your toes while sitting down with your legs outstretched in front of you, due to a tight lower back or even tighter hamstrings? Usually when trying to force yourself into a position like this you expose the vulnerable knee and hip joints to extreme resistance, resulting in limited motion and possibly pain. Rather than forcing your legs and lower back into this compromising position, sneak up on the movement by first bending your knees slightly and slowly lowering your upper body over your bent knees. From there gradually lower your legs out straight and relax into the stretch until you have reached your maximum position at that moment in time. This is how to overcome some of your earlier limitations when stretching these muscle groups, and by using the above *StretchSmart* method you can improve on your flexibility without struggling. This is just one of many examples of how you will learn an easier approach to becoming more supple.

HOW DOES STRETCHING PREVENT INJURY?

One of the greatest benefits of stretching is that you're able to increase the length of both your muscles and tendons to a certain degree. This leads to an increased range of movement, which means your limbs and joints can move farther before an injury occurs. Let's take a look at a few examples.

If your neck muscles are tight and stiff, this will limit your ability to look behind you, or turn your head as far as you would like. If for some reason your head is jerked to the side, past its normal range of movement, for example, this could result in a muscle tear or strain related to a sport or auto accident. You can help to prevent this from happening by increasing the flexibility, and the range of movement, of the muscles and tendons in your neck.

And what about the muscles in the back of your legs? The hamstring muscles, these muscles are put under a huge strain when you are participating in any sort of sport that involves running. Short, tight hamstring muscles can spell disaster for many sports athletes. By ensuring these muscles are loose and flexible, you'll cut your chances of a hamstring injury dramatically. You may have heard it said that an athlete has "thrown out a shoulder"? While only a true dislocation could do this, the expression is most likely referring to a strained shoulder that has been overused and gone beyond the normal range of motion one too many times, resulting in an injury. You will learn how not to incur these types of injuries by using the *StretchSmart* movements to provide flexibility in every possible angle to enhance your muscles' abilities.

How else can stretching help? While injuries can occur at any time, they are more likely to occur if the muscles are fatigued, tight and depleted of energy. Fatigued, tight muscles are also less capable of performing the skills required for your particular sport or activity. Stretching can help to prevent an injury by promoting recovery and decreasing soreness. Stretching ensures that your muscles and tendons are in good working order. The more conditioned your muscles and tendons are, the better they can handle the rigors of a sport and exercises, and it's less likely that they'll become injured.

So as you can see, there's more to stretching than most people think. Stretching is a simple and effective activity that will help you to enhance your athletic performance, decrease your likelihood of sports injury and minimize muscle soreness.

While warming-up is important, a good cool-down also plays a vital role in helping to prevent sports injury. How? A good cool-down will prevent blood from pooling in your limbs. It will also prevent waste products, such as lactic acid, from building up in your muscles. Not only that, a good cool-down will help your muscles and tendons relax and loosen, stopping them from becoming stiff and tight. Allowing more time at the end of your workouts to stretch out your muscles will improve your flexibility dramatically.

TYPES OF STRETCHING

Now that you know why stretching is important, let's examine different types of stretching techniques and their uniqueness, as well as how you can utilize this information to improve your flexibility and enhance your workouts.

As a general rule the following stretches are categorized into groups of stretching. Stretches are either dynamic—meaning they involve motion, or static—meaning they involve no motion. The thought was that dynamic stretches affect active flexibility and static stretches affect fixed flexibility. As research techniques improved, we learned more about fast and slow switches, fibers, and the role of the Golgi tendon, to trick the muscles into relaxing. That is where *StretchSmart* comes into play, utilizing both methods to increase further range of motion in your muscles with the least resistance when doing the stretches, thus providing the benefit of better flexibility without the boredom of holding a position for a prolonged period of time, but more on that later. First, let's look at the variations of stretching categories.

THE DIFFERENT TYPES OF STRETCHING ARE:
- Ballistic stretching
- Dynamic stretching
- Active stretching
- Passive (or relaxed) stretching
- Static stretching
- Isometric stretching
- PNF stretching
- Ballistic Stretching

Ballistic stretching uses the momentum of a moving body or a limb in an attempt to force it beyond its normal range of motion. This is stretching by bouncing into a stretched position, using the stretched muscles like a rubber band that pulls you out of the stretched position. An example would be bending over and bouncing down repeatedly to try to touch your toes with your hands. This type of stretching is not considered helpful and can lead to injury for most people who try to do it. It does not allow your muscles to adjust to, and relax into, the stretch. It may instead cause your muscles to tighten up by repeatedly activating the Golgi tendon reflex response at the joint muscle, resulting in more soreness than necessary to increase your flexibility.

DYNAMIC STRETCHING

Dynamic stretching involves moving parts of your body and gradually increasing range and speed of movement, or both. Do not confuse dynamic stretching with ballistic stretching. Dynamic stretching consists of controlled leg and arm movements that take you gently to the limits of your range of motion. Ballistic stretches involve trying to force a part of the body beyond its range of motion. In dynamic stretches, there are no bounces or "jerky" movements and these types of stretches make up the bulk of *StretchSmart* program. Dynamic stretching improves dynamic flexibility and is a complete workout in itself but also quite useful as part of your warm-up for any workout you may have planned after stretching.

ACTIVE STRETCHING

Active stretching is also referred to as static-active stretching. An active stretch is one where you assume a position and then hold it there with no assistance. Learning to incorporate your muscle groups as a unit is by far more effective and less painful, as shown in *StretchSmart* principle used throughout this book. For example, while standing, bring your leg up high above your waistline in front of you and then hold it there without using anything to rest on or hold on to other than your leg muscles themselves, to keep the leg in that extended position. The tension of the antagonists (opposing muscles) is an active stretch that helps to relax the muscles being stretched by the antagonist muscles. Thus, you are stretching more muscle groups with one movement rather than using many stretches to accomplish the same effect, while enhancing your balance and strength as well.

Active stretching increases active flexibility and strengthens your antagonistic muscles as a unit of activity rather than isolating one particular muscle. Thus, you rarely have to hold these stretches for prolonged periods of time to benefit from the stretch being performed. These are fun and challenging stretches done throughout your routine to keep your body temperature up and your core strong.

PASSIVE STRETCHING

Passive stretching is also referred to as relaxed stretching. A passive stretch is one where you assume a position and hold it with some other part of your body, or with the assistance of a partner or some other apparatus. For example, using the wall to support yourself as you move from one stretch to the next or doing the splits with your legs while sitting down is anther passive stretch by using the floor as resistance to maintain your position. You will learn how to use the floor, wall, chair, towel and anything else you can think of to help improve your flexibility, which is easier than straining into and holding a position.

Slow, relaxed stretching is useful in relieving muscle spasms due to an injury. Passive stretching is also very good for "cooling down" after a workout and helps slow down your heart rate and breathing while reducing post-workout muscle soreness and fatigue.

STATIC STRETCHING

Many people assume passive stretching is static stretching. However, there is a distinction between the two and it's key to your flexibility workouts.

Static stretching involves holding a position. That is, you stretch to the farthest point and hold the stretch.

Passive stretching is a technique in which you are relaxed and make no further efforts to increase the range of motion. Instead, using external forces such as the wall or towel creates an outside driving force to improve your motion with minimum exertion.

ISOMETRIC OR RESISTANCE STRETCHING

Isometric stretching is a type of static stretching that involves the resistance of muscle groups through isometric contractions or tensing of your stretched muscles .The use of isometric stretching is one method to develop increased static-passive flexibility and combined with dynamic and active stretching will speed up your flexibility as opposed to doing any of these types of stretches alone.

Isometric stretches also help to develop strength in your "tensed" muscle groups that helps to develop your flexibility.

The most common ways to provide the needed resistance for an isometric stretch are to apply resistance manually to one's own limbs, or to have a partner apply the resistance, or to use an apparatus such as a wall, chair, towel or the floor to provide resistance.

An example of manual resistance would be holding onto the ball of your foot to keep it from flexing while you are using the muscles of your calf to try and straighten your instep so that the toes are pointed.

An example of using the wall to provide resistance is, while you attempt to force your back against the wall, you tilt your pelvis; this is another example that will be explained in a later chapter.

Isometric stretching is not recommended for children whose bones are still growing. This age group is usually already flexible enough that the strong stretches produced by the isometric contraction have a much higher risk of damaging tendons and connective tissue. It is also not for individuals who have had surgery on a joint in the muscle region; in this case the active and passive stretches would be better.

HOW RESISTANCE STRETCHING WORKS

The science behind resistance training is fairly straight forward and once you understand why your body responds in this way, the more stretches you can create to improve your motion. When a muscle is contracted, some of the fibers contract, not all, only enough to get the job done. As you increase the load on the muscles, you will increase the use of more muscle fibers. Similarly, when your muscles are stretched, some of your fibers are elongated and some remain inactive.

During an isometric contraction, some of your muscle fibers in the stretched position, or resting position, are being pulled upon from both ends by the muscles that are contracting. The result is that those resting fibers become stretched as well.

The effectiveness of the isometric exercise occurs when your muscle group that is already in a stretched position is subjected to an isometric contraction. In this case, some of the muscle fibers are already stretched before the contraction, and, if held long enough, the initial passive stretch overcomes the Golgi reflex response and triggers the lengthening reaction, inhibiting the stretched fibers from contracting. When the isometric contraction is relaxed and the contracting fibers returned to their resting length, the stretched fibers retain their ability to stretch beyond their past range of motion, before the stretch. The whole muscle group will be able to stretch beyond its initial maximum, and you will have increased your flexibility.

While you may not understand completely how the mechanism works, you will be able to feel the difference in your muscles after applying these methods in your workout.

PNF STRETCHING

PNF stretching is currently the more popular stretching style seen in professional sports today to increase flexibility. Unfortunately, when people try to pick up this technique they use it more as a bouncing method that, as we discussed earlier, can lead to injuries quickly if done improperly. Often this stretch is done with a partner and you need to put a lot of trust in that person not to cause you injury in the process and to offer enough resistance to get results. A tricky situation I'd rather not be in, nor should you. Instead I will explain what it is first then how you will be able to use this method in your *StretchSmart* routine to enhance your flexibility.

PNF is an acronym for proprioceptive neuromuscular facilitation. This stretching technique combines passive stretching and isometric stretching in order to achieve maximum flexibility in your muscles. These post-isometric relaxation-stretching techniques are when a muscle group is passively stretched, then contracted isometrically against resistance (a partner or wall) while in a stretched position, and then passively stretched again through the resulting increased range of motion.

Some PNF techniques also employ isometric antagonist contraction where the antagonists of the stretched muscles are contracted. This hold and relax drill is effective in overcoming tight muscles groups that normally do not respond to other stretching techniques.

Like isometric stretching, PNF stretching is also not recommended for children whose bones are still growing or a person who has had surgery to a muscle or joint region being stretched.

HOW PNF WORKS

Remember that during an isometric stretch, when the muscle performing the isometric contraction is relaxed, it retains its ability to stretch beyond its initial resting maximum length. PNF tries to take immediate advantage of this increased range of motion by immediately subjecting the contracted muscle to a passive stretch.

This stretching technique uses the period of time immediately following the isometric contraction to train the stretched Golgi tendon receptors to get used to this new, increased, range of muscle length.

Most people wait too late to start a stretching program, usually after they have sustained an injury and are seeking professional advice for their injuries and in most cases are given stretches to perform to help speed their recovery back to health.

As you can see there is a number of ways to stretch your muscles besides bending over at your waist and hanging there trying to touch your toes. The stretching you will do as you incorporate the above stretching styles in your *StretchSmart* routine will help you prevent injuries from occurring in muscle groups that are too tight, as well as prevent you from overstraining while improving your flexibility and your overall range of motion and health. Now let's move on to the next chapter and discuss how you should start off in accomplishing a better stretching program for a more supple and stronger body.

STRETCHING—SCIENTIFICALLY?

WHAT ABOUT STUDIES THAT SAY STRETCHING DOES NOT PREVENT INJURIES?

Most of the studies I've reviewed attempt to determine the effects of stretching on injury prevention. Stretching, by itself, will not prevent injury. In fact, stretching can cause injury if certain precautions aren't taken.

Plus, it's not just a flexibility problem that can lead to injury.

It could be:

- A strength imbalance, when one side of your body is stronger than the other

- Instability or balance issues

- Postural imbalances

- A physical imbalance, such as one leg length longer than the other

Stretching is one very important component that assists in reducing the risk of injury. The best results are achieved when stretching is used in combination with other injury reduction techniques.

Stretching and its effect on physical performance and injury prevention is something that can't be measured scientifically. The effects of stretching are difficult to measure and all the studies that I have seen are nothing more than anecdotal.

You see, stretching is not a science. It is nearly impossible to prove anything about stretching, scientifically. Sure, you can measure the effect of stretching on flexibility with simple tests like the "Sit and Reach" test, but then to determine how that affects athletic performance or injury susceptibility is, again, nearly impossible. So while studies are beneficial for learning about how your muscles function in a given parameter, it's best to focus on how you feel and move during your stretching routine to improve your flexibility.

STRETCH REFLEX

When a muscle is placed into a stretch, the muscle spindle inside the muscle belly records the change in length and sends signals to the spine, which conveys this information to your brain. This triggers the stretch reflex, which attempts to resist the change in muscle length by causing the stretched muscle to contract. The more sudden the change in muscle length, the stronger the muscle contractions will be. This basic function of the muscle spindle helps to maintain muscle tone and to protect your body from injury.

One of the reasons for holding a stretch for a prolonged period of time is that as you hold the muscle in a stretched position, the muscle spindle in theory becomes accustomed to the new length and reduces its signaling to contract your muscles. Gradually, your muscle's stretch receptors adapt to the lengthening of your muscles due to the stretches.

MUSCLE GOLGI TENDON REACTION

When your muscles contract, tension is produced at the point where the muscle is connected to the tendon, where the Golgi tendon is located. The Golgi tendon records the change in tension, and the rate of change of the tension, and sends signals to the brain to convey this information. When this tension exceeds a certain threshold, it triggers the lengthening reaction that inhibits your muscles from contracting and causes them to relax. This basic function of the Golgi tendon helps to protect the muscles, tendons, and ligaments from injury. The lengthening reaction is possible only because the signaling of the Golgi tendon to the brain is powerful enough to overcome the signaling of the muscle spindles telling the muscle to contract.

For this reason you will learn how to use resistance to enhance this lengthening reaction to occur, thus helping your muscles to relax into the stretches.

CHAPTER SUMMARY

WHY WE STRETCH AND THE BENEFITS OF DOING SO:

- Stretching is key to preventing injuries due to lack of motion

- You will improve your range of motion

- The advantage of more flexibility is stronger muscles working at full capacity

- You will improve your circulation

- You will restore optimum body function, providing ease in your body's movement and everyday activity

- You will help minimize muscle soreness

- You will build up your muscle capacity to withstand your other training exercises

- You will prevent stiffness and improve your body's bio-mechanics

- Stretching should not hurt

- Keeping hydrated when performing stretches will help prevent muscle aches

- There are many variations to stretching and you'll learn to use them all to improve your comprehensive flexibility

CHAPTER 2

STIFF AS A BOARD?
PROTOCOL FOR EASING INTO IT.

This chapter was created for all those individuals who think they can't stretch no matter how hard they try and fail to completely stretch out their bodies. It is also for those who want to improve their flexibility by enhancing their efforts.

Let's address some concerns about your limitations and when to stretch before dealing with the recommended protocols for improving your flexibility.

BEYOND STRUCTURAL LIMITATIONS

Are there "normal" ranges of flexible motion for everyone? Not really, there are only guidelines based on the general population and their guidelines do not take into account past injuries to joints, ligaments, muscles or bone fractures. Don't worry if you don't fit into a certain category when it comes to your flexibility. The only one you should be competing with is yourself.

So you never could touch the floor when bending over at the waist while standing—this doesn't mean you can't improve on your muscle flexibility by outsmarting some shortcomings in your structure, such as long legs and shorter arms or a longer torso and shorter legs, disproportional body parts will not slow your progress during *StretchSmart* program.

Using *StretchSmart*, you'll be able to overcome these barriers and improve your flexibility and the way you feel with new and improved range of motion. You'll be able to notice this in a shorter period of time than with traditional reach-and-hold stretches.

How far you travel within a given joint and muscle range determines your flexibility, while being able to travel through the whole range without pain is key and always desirable. This chapter will teach you how to accomplish that in the shortest period of time using science and relaxation techniques to enhance your flexibility regardless of how stiff you are now.

WARM-UP BEFORE STRETCHING?

This by far is the most typical question I get from my patients and clients at seminars. I have a two-part answer. First, what time of year is it for you? Is it warm where you live year round? Or do you have four seasons? Okay, let's narrow this down: when it's hot, like in the summer, your body temperature is elevated to start with and you need less motion to work up a sweat, and overall, your joints are not nearly as tight as in the middle of the winter. If it's winter time and very cold, it will take you longer to warm up your body's temperature. A good idea in the wintertime is to wear layers so you can take off clothes as you begin to sweat. As a general rule, warm muscles are much more easily stretched than cold muscles.

Always warm-up first to get your blood circulating throughout your body and especially in the muscle groups. A warm-up should be slow and rhythmic, addressing the larger muscle groups first before moving onto the smaller muscles. There is no set time to accomplish a warm-up. You can go through this sequence of exercises below to warm up your entire body.

EXAMPLE OF WARMING UP BEFORE STRETCHING
- Walking 10 to 15 minutes at an easy pace with some arm swinging
- Riding a bicycle.
- A few push-ups against a wall
- Body weight half squats
- Body weight lunges
- Calf raises
- Warm-up at a low intensity

This provides the body with a period of adjustment between rest and activity. Once you have warmed up and broken a light sweat you are now ready to do your stretching exercises.

STRETCH BEFORE AND AFTER CARDIO-RELATED EXERCISING

I recommend stretching both before, during and after exercising, each for different reasons. Stretching before an activity (after the warm-up) improves your range of motion and reduces the chance of injury. Stretching during a workout helps keep your muscles supple and more responsive. Stretching after exercise ensures your muscles will relax and facilitate your normal resting muscle length to joint and tissue structures, and most importantly aid in the removal of unwanted waste products, thus reducing muscle soreness and stiffness.

STRETCH DURING YOUR WEIGHTLIFTING WORKOUTS

Both strength training and flexibility training are so important. Those of you who have a hard time finding time to incorporate two different types of workouts into your routine can combine your stretching with your strength training programs. If you have had any experience in strength training, you know that for each exercise and muscle group you train, you have a certain number of sets, usually between two and three.

Between each set, you need to rest and let your muscles recover before going on to the next set. Well, what better use of your time than to stretch the muscles that you're currently training and the muscles around them?

STRETCHING PRINCIPLES AND GUIDELINES

When done correctly, stretching can prevent injuries, increase your range of motion, promote relaxation, improve athletic performance and improve your posture, reduce your stress and keep your body feeling loose and agile. Use these guidelines to get the most out of your *StretchSmart* program.

NO BOUNCING
I am still amazed to see people bouncing or more like jerking themselves into positions, tensing their muscles into a stretch. Not only is this counterproductive but dangerous too. All too often I hear someone tell me they pulled their back or hamstring trying to stretch out. This of course will happen over and over again if you try to launch yourself beyond your muscles' and body's ability by using fast-paced motion, which only further triggers the body's protective mechanism to fire off at the joint and muscle junction. This bouncing process will just slow down your progress. Rather, *StretchSmart* exercises will keep you going through one contin-

uous loop of movements, improving your range of motion without fits of jerking, or stop-and-holds, to accomplish greater flexibility.

TEMPO

Similar to the drawbacks of bouncing, you do not want to go too fast through your stretches nor do you want to hold on forever in one particular position. You want to set a tempo to your movement patterns with a rhythmic pace that allows you enough time to feel the stretch while keeping your breathing even and allowing your body to warm up gradually. Each person is different and I can only give you guidelines to follow—it has to feel right to you.

DO NOT REACH BEYOND YOUR LIMITS

When you bring your arms forward, reaching over your legs while sitting, there are no markers to say where your hands should end up, so why make it a goal to grab your feet and hold them? Rather, feel your muscles lengthening; your body will let you know the right length to reach for. Don't compromise your posture and your joints and muscle integrity to just go a little further. With all your stretches, get into a comfortable zone and feel your muscles stretching rather than pulling due to an exertion.

DO NOT HYPER-EXTEND

Since hyper-extended joints are basically a problem of too-loose ligaments and tendons around the regions commonly located in the wrists, elbows and knee, you can cause or exacerbate such looseness through poor alignment in your stretching routine. The soft tissues at risk of being overstretched include your ligaments deep inside the joints. There are also several large tendons that normally help prevent hyper-extension from occurring but for whatever reason they are not. If you fall into this category you need to pay close attention to the way your muscles feel during the movements and not go beyond your joint integrity. *StretchSmart* exercises will help stabilize your joints by strengthening the surrounding muscles while improving your flexibility.

USE PROPER POSTURE ALIGNMENT

We have all been told since we were children to sit and stand up straight. Posture has been considered important for our health and our image, but it is also very important to our stretching ability as well. Staying supple rather than rigid, when moving into one position and the next, will help you tremendously by improving your range of motion, and by not allowing your spine to tighten up while you move. Keeping your core strong will affect your flexibility and endurance in sustaining the positions you wish to achieve.

STRETCH YOUR MUSCLES AS A UNIT NOT AS ONE INDIVIDUAL MUSCLE AT A TIME

Commonly you will isolate a particular muscle group, let's say the quadriceps—the muscles on top of your thighs—by standing and pulling your ankle back behind your hip and holding it there for a few seconds then repeating with the opposite leg. Did you really work only the front of your thighs with that stretch? It takes the hip flexors in front of your thighs to relax and your hip extensor-glutes to relax for you to stretch the quads. A more productive method of stretching allows you to stretch all three major groups like they were intended to move, because they work as a unit. For example, they work together when you walk or jog or go up a flight of stairs. *StretchSmart* exercises allow you to stretch more muscle groups with a single movement, making your stretching routine more efficient and more productive in improving your flexibility in a shorter period of time.

EXERCISE ORDER

One of the most effective ways to stretch is to do so in a certain order to thoroughly warm-up and stretch muscles that you are going to use in the next movement so your muscles will work together, rather than stretching one particular muscle group then moving on to the next and so on. The old theory of working your bigger muscle groups does not hold true for *StretchSmart* stretches. Rather, the pattern of stretches will allow you to open up your range of motion in your muscles as they warm up, allowing more flexibility into the muscles as they are lengthening with greater range. By stretching synergistic muscle groups, you will actually stretch several muscles and the benefit of this is that you are able to better stretch by using the supporting muscles to help increase your flexibility in a particular movement.

Ideally, by organizing the exercises within your stretching routine, you minimize the effort required to perform your routine, and maximize the effectiveness of your stretching time.

BREATHING
WHY IS BREATHING SO IMPORTANT WHEN DOING STRETCHING?

Simply put, you unconsciously breathe at the rate in which your body uses energy. For example, when you start to jog from a walk your lungs adjust to the load and the need to supply your muscles the desirable level of oxygen that is required to complete the task. It only becomes an issue when you try to force yourself to breathe a certain way and you end up holding your breath or forcing out too much air, causing your body to tighten up when you should be relaxed while stretching. What exactly are you tightening up, you might wonder? It's your diaphragm and the surrounding muscles in the abdominal and back muscles. When you breathe out, the diaphragm contracts to move your lungs up, thus causing your lungs to be contracted and lowering the pressure in your lungs. When you inhale, the diaphragm muscles relax down and allow your lungs to expand and fill up with more air.

PROPER BREATHING CONTROL

Proper breathing is important for successful stretching. Proper breathing helps to relax your body, increases blood flow throughout your muscles, and helps to mechanically remove lactic acid and other by-products out of the muscle region. You should be taking slow, relaxed breaths when you stretch, trying to exhale as the muscle is lengthening and inhaling when changing positions or resting.

Breathe in slowly through your nose, expanding your diaphragm, not lifting or sticking out your chest, and then exhale slowly through the nose.
Inhaling through the nose has several purposes, including cleaning the air and insuring proper temperature and humidity for oxygen transfer into the lungs. The breath should be natural and the diaphragm and abdomen should remain soft. You should not force your breathing.

The rate of breathing should be based on the overall exertion of the movement. Allow your body to adapt to the new position and relax into the stretch, while also relaxing your breathing as you move into each new position.

STRETCH YOUR POSTURAL MUSCLES DAILY

Making sure your postural muscles are supple throughout the day will improve the stretching of the rest of your muscles. These muscle groups become fatigued due to our static positions of sitting throughout the day hunched over a computer or driving in a car. In the next chapter you will learn how easy it is to stretch out these important muscle groups and how doing so will improve your range of motion.

RELAX

As I discussed above, the importance of breathing is reflected in your ability to relax while you stretch. It does sound like common sense but it is so easy to self-sabotage yourself by tensing and holding your breath or flexing muscles that should be relaxed. Take a few minutes to clear your mind before stretching; listening to relaxing music while stretching can help you further decompress to improve your flexibility.

DON'T COMPETE

Since childhood, I have had the fortunate opportunity of training with some of the best competitive martial arts athletes and now see many professional and amateur athletes in my center. What they all have in common is the desire to win, and so they are driven in their workouts. Unfortunately, many end up injured now and then and many still neglect the practice of stretching properly. They choose to be aggressive even while stretching when they should be as relaxed as possible, allowing their bodies to conform to the stretch rather than be forced into a position.

BODY MECHANICS

Proper body mechanics cannot be overemphasized when you are stretching or performing any other form of exercise. Being limp as a rag doll is just as bad as being rigid when performing your stretches. It's important to find that groove in between where you are in control of all your muscle groups throughout the duration of the movement.

VARIATIONS

Throughout this book you will be instructed to perform movements in a certain order and way that you may not be able to achieve right away. The instructions should be used as a reference and not an end point of a completed movement. You may feel more comfortable supporting yourself on your forearms rather than your hands to feel the stretch more effectively. By all means, go ahead, do what works best for your body type and the state of your flexibility at that moment in time. Some movement will be offered with a number of ways to perform the stretch with similar results or to further enhance your range of motion with a slight variation.

PATIENCE

The flexibility progress is usually so gradual that you won't notice a day-to-day improvement. It's more likely that after a few weeks, you'll look back and realize that your stiffness has decreased and you are able to move more freely than when you first started this program. As you improve you will become less sensitive to a particular movement and you'll breathe easier during the action as well.

DO NO HARM

Don't try to force yourself into a position or stretch out hard all your muscles at once in a given workout period. Gradually build up to the amount of time it takes you to complete the movements. Don't rush into the program. Being overly sore because you are pushing too hard will just slow your progress to becoming more supple.

SETS AND REPS

These are general guidelines for you to follow. If you are unable to complete the entire recommended workout, don't fret. Use them as short and long term goals toward your progress in achieving the best flexibility you can during any given workout. Hold times if any are given with the description of the exercises in the proceeding chapters. Your rest periods between repetitions and sets should be treated like those in any of your other workouts except that you will be resting less to maintain your body's temperature elevation to keep your muscles loose.

A note about intensity levels in your workouts. Intensity is usually used on some type of pain scale. Instead I want you to think more of the number of times you perform the movement and how long it takes you to recover before moving onto the next exercise. For example, it takes you ten minutes to do your wall stretches and you still feel you have plenty of energy left to go through them again. This would be considered a light intensity workout. While doing an intermediate workout, you may feel fairly tired after going through a set of exercises and need more energy to do them again. You get the idea. Based on your own personal energy levels, the exercise is light if you still have something left to give in your workouts, and advanced if you are ready to hit the showers and be done with your workout.

BEGINNER LEVEL 1

- Light intensity
- Three times per week
- Rest days
- Two times per week or more
- Duration
- 20 to 25 minutes per workout

BEGINNER LEVEL 2

- Light intensity
- Two times per week
- Medium intensity
- One time per week
- Rest days
- Three times per week or more
- Duration
- 20 to 25 minutes per workout

INTERMEDIATE LEVEL 1

- Light intensity
- Two times per week
- Medium intensity
- Two times per week
- Rest days
- Two times per week or more
- Duration
- 25 to 30 minutes per workout

INTERMEDIATE LEVEL 2

- Light intensity
- Two times per week
- Medium intensity
- One time per week
- Rest days
- Three times per week or more
- Duration
- 20 to 25 minutes per workout

ADVANCED LEVEL

- Light intensity
- Two times per week
- Medium intensity
- Two times per week
- Hard intensity
- One time per week, followed by a rest or light workout the next day
- Rest days
- One time per week or more
- Duration
- 40 to 50 minutes per workout

As you can see you have a wide variety of ways to change your workouts around to suit the way you feel each day and how you are improving your flexibility. Note the way you get up in the morning and walk around—are you stiff and sore at first and then you loosen up as you move more? Or is the soreness consistent throughout the day after your workout? Being aware of how your body moves over the next couple weeks and months will help you learn more about yourself and your thresholds, as you break through to achieve greater range of motion and flexibility in areas you thought were impossible until now.

Now let's move on to the next chapter and focus on those important-to-your-posture muscle groups to enhance your flexibility and get into your routine for stretching your body and improving the way you feel and move.

CHAPTER SUMMARY

- No bouncing
- Do not overreach beyond your limits
- Use proper posture alignment
- Stretch your postural muscles daily
- Stretch your muscles as a unit
- Variations
- Patience

CHAPTER 3

PERFECT POSTURE—
BEYOND STRUCTURAL LIMITATIONS
AND IMPROVING HOW YOU LOOK

WHAT IS PERFECT POSTURE AND
HOW DO YOU GET IT?

Why do you need it anyway? What are the benefits of good posture? We have always been told to sit and stand up straight since we were children. Posture has been considered important for our health and image, but what is perfect posture? How do you compare it from one individual to the next? I'll tell you clearly that it is not about sitting like a board in a rigid position staring straight ahead in an uncomfortable position with your back muscles tight and your shoulders thrown back.

First let's look at your own posture and see how it not only affects your image and how you feel but also how it influences your range of motion. You can't stretch out your muscles if you hold yourself in an improper position when you are not exercising.

Poor posture not only affects your muscle flexibility, it also makes you look older, shorter and heavier as well. Beside the appearance, your health is affected by poor posture, by its causing your breathing to be forced and labor-intensive, and compressing your spine and weakening your core in the process.

A LOOK IN THE MIRROR

What is the first thing about your posture that you notice when you stand in front of a full length mirror?
- Any head tilt to the right or the left when you look straight ahead?
- Does your chin drop to one side, right or left?
- Does one ear appear higher than the other?
- Is one shoulder higher than the other?
- Are one or both shoulders rounded forward?
- Do your hands rest out to the side or is one hand turned in more than the other?

- Do you stand with both legs squared off shoulder width apart or is one leg in front of the other?
- Do you shift your weight onto one foot more than the other?
- Are your knees turned out or one leg turned in?
- Are your feet positioned straight ahead or are they turned out or in?

Take notes on what you see and come back to them in a few weeks after using *StretchSmart* exercises. You will be able to see changes in your posture and be able to use the mirror as your gauge as to how your flexibility is improving and how you are progressing.

Now let's move on to the side view of your posture.

SIDE VIEW IN THE MIRROR

From the side you may want to have someone take a picture or if you have two mirrors nearby you can see by yourself.

- Is your head sticking forward away from your shoulders? How far, one inch or two?
- Does your chin jut out and down from your body?
- Are your shoulders rounded forward?
- Do you have an overemphasized roundness to your upper back? A hump?
- Does your lower back region have a sway in it? An overemphasized curve?
- Is one shoulder higher than the other when compared side to side?
- Is your hip turned out more on one side or the other?

Again write down what you observe. You will come back to these observations in a few weeks and see for yourself how your body can change with the proper stretching exercises that will make you look taller, younger and thinner.

IDENTIFYING INCORRECT POSTURE

Before we dive into what are good posture positions, let's look at some common, stress-inducing postural positions you may find yourself in, as the above clues are the results of these stressors placed on your body day in and day out. To improve upon your posture you must first identify what needs improvement by examining your own postural habits throughout the day, such as:

- Standing and waiting in a line.
- Sitting at your desk at work.
- While driving or riding in a bus or train.
- While carrying a backpack or suitcase.
- Carrying grocery or shopping bags.
- Watching TV—that favorite couch or chair may not be doing any wonders for your posture.

At regular intervals during the day, take a moment to make a note of your posture and at what time of the day your posture changes. Also take note of others around you: first thing in the morning, do you notice people standing more upright and attentive in meetings compared to late afternoon? Do you notice more slouching and more people dragging around near the end of a typical day? It's happening all around you.

EXAMPLES OF POOR POSTURE AND STRESSES

The following are examples of common pitfalls of poor ergonomics and bad postural habits that you need to be aware of if you want to improve upon your posture and your overall flexibility, to improve the way you feel and move.

- Wearing high-heel shoes.
- Not using your headrest in your car.
- Slouching forward with your head down.
- Not using the back of your chair for proper support.
- Looking down too much when walking.
- Working for prolonged periods at a time in front of the computer without re-positioning your head.
- Carrying something heavy on one side of your body day in and day out, like a laptop, purse, or backpack.
- Cradling a phone between your neck and shoulder.
- Watching TV from the same location every time you do so.
- Sleeping on a pillow that is more than three years old.
- Sleeping on a worn-out mattress that does not offer you the right amount of support.

These are just a few major repeated episodes that occur in your daily life that cause a decrease in your range of motion and can be the causes of chronic stiffness and pain, too. Now let's look in more detail at each commonly held position and see how it affects your body's ability to move. This will also give you a better understanding of how to free yourself up to move around more easily.

BAD POSTURAL SITTING POSITIONS

- Slumping forward away from the chair for support, restricting your ribcage, thus using more effort to breathe properly.
- Leaning forward and resting your weight on your thighs rather than your spine, causing your leg muscles to tighten and shorten your hip flexors in your legs, causing a pull on your already stressed body.
- Slouching forward down into the seat while just supporting the head or shoulders only, causing undue stress on your spine. This gravitational stress to the spine causes an increased load on the muscles that compensate for the spinal misalignment, causing further muscle and spinal stiffness.
- Tucking one leg underneath your other leg while sitting.
- Dropping your head forward.
- Weakening the core while not maintaining abdominal pressure, which supports your vital organs.
- The source of much pain and discomfort in your neck and back regions.

The ideal sitting posture puts far less strain on your neck, shoulders, back and hamstrings. The 'forced' and 'slouched' postures require more muscular effort than balanced sitting.

In this composed sitting position your posture allows for proper and relaxed breathing because the spine is supporting the weight of your head into the chair and enabling your ribs to move freely without the above constraints. Your core is strong and your lower back is supported against the chair.

Remember to change positions or get up and move around every twenty minutes or so to help keep your muscles and joints supple. When you do get stuck sitting for long periods at a time and are unable to get up, for example, during an airplane flight or when sitting in a movie theater, try to sit with the full weight of your upper body on your buttocks and thighs.

Good posture is important to transmit those loads appropriately. Maintaining that neutral spinal position when everything is supported equally throughout your body will help prevent stiffness and promote better posture while sitting.

HERE ARE A FEW MORE TIPS TO PUT INTO ACTION WHILE YOU SIT.

- Position your feet flat on the floor or on a book or box to keep your legs parallel to the floor. If your chair is too tall for you and there is no way to lower it to the floor without your being able to do your work then simply stack books or a box under your feet to bring your legs parallel to the floor, thus putting less stress on your spine and entire core region.
- Position your back and shoulders against the chair.
- Position your elbows and lower arms to rest on the armrests if you have them.
- Keep your shoulders relaxed, not pulled back tightly nor rounded forward.

If you have a difficult time getting your lower back against the back of the chair in this position you can roll up a towel and place it behind your lower back for support until you become more flexible and stronger in your core.

STANDING POSTURE

Standing position requires very different muscle groups to interface and just plain rebel against each other to accomplish such poor posture over a long period of time. Like sitting, standing in a neutral relaxed position requires less muscle involvement to maintain the proper balance in your body.

When you were told to stand up straight as a child, what did you do? Did you, like the majority of people do, tighten your lower back, suck in your stomach, stick out your chest and keep your arms stiff by your side with your chin pointing upward? This "attention" position shows the most common response when you ask someone to stand up straight. On the other hand, have you ever thought that if you knew what proper posture was, you would already be standing correctly? How do you suddenly know to stand properly if you have not done it for years? In place of jerking yourself up to the position of standing straight, you'll teach your body to relax in a neutral position with your muscles at ease after stretching them with the customized *StretchSmart* sequence of exercises, which will increase your postural muscles' flexibility and strengthen your core at the same time. In a short time slouching will feel uncomfortable to you.

SLEEPING
MATTRESS

Does your back hurt when you wake up each morning? How old is your mattress? More than ten years? Your mattress may be too soft. As a general rule, firm surfaces usually provide better back and neck support.

PILLOW
Next, check your pillow. Does it help you maintain a straight line from ear to shoulder, the proper alignment you learned from standing properly? If not, you may need to go shopping for a pillow.

POOR SLEEPING HABITS
- Sleeping on your stomach.
- Sleeping with your head turned the same direction every night while lying on your stomach.
- Sleeping only on one side.
- Sleeping on two or more pillows.

To correct these habits and improve your sleep as well as rest your muscles and joints so they are less stiff and you are more relaxed with more energy from a restful slumber, try taking these steps.
- Rotate your mattress from head to toe every even calendar month and flip your mattress over on the odd months. You will add years to the use of your bed and not sleep in your own body's groove night after night, allowing more restful sleep and more relaxed muscles.
- Get rid of saggy mattresses, as they cause back and neck strain.
- Buy a pillow every two or three years or sooner if you notice your head is sagging down when you lie on your side.
- Place a pillow behind your knees when you are lying on your back.
- Place a pillow between your knees when you lie on your side.

HOW TO IMPROVE YOUR POSTURE
GET YOUR HEAD ON STRAIGHT

Spinal alignment is so important for perfect posture, and neck and back comfort. Thus we will address the anterior head lean position.

A head that hangs too far forward is the most widespread posture misalignment problem, and one that causes far more problems than you might think in today's society with computer use, and sitting for hours in a static position while commuting for hours. The reason is that a head is heavy. The average human head weights between 11 to 14 pounds, the same as a bowling ball!

Your head is supposed to rest directly over the shoulders in the body's center of gravity. When it hangs forward even slightly it is no longer in the center of gravity, and the muscles in the neck and upper back have to work harder just to hold your head up. The farther your head is held in front of your shoulders the more strain on your neck and upper back muscles.

This starts a vicious chain reaction down the entire spine, thus inhibiting your overall range of motion and flexibility.

We will discuss the proper alignment of your head over your spine with specific exercises to correct the forward lean through simple but very effective means.

YOUR POSTURAL ANATOMY
TRAPS

The upper back muscles are made up of many muscle groups that support your head and help stabilize the region as a whole. If one side is out of balance with the other the result can throw off your entire spinal balance, giving you tight muscles and stiff joints.

The trapezius muscle is a large, diamond-shaped muscle that runs from the base of your head out to your posterior shoulder muscles and down your mid-back, ending at your last ribs near your lower back. A very large muscle group for sure, and a major work horse when it comes to your upper and mid-back posture and flexibility.

When your head juts forward and down, your upper trap fibers are constantly under tension to hold the weight of your head (the bowling ball weight) in the wrong position. Over a period of time, your traps become tight and reduce your range of motion in your neck by inhibiting the upward and downward motion of your head.

This constant tension brings on numerous ailments from tension headaches, to pain in the neck.

LEVATORS

These side muscles run along the sides of the traps and attach to the upper shoulder region. When irritated, this muscle group triggers pain into the shoulder, arm and even the hands when flexibility is lost in this muscle group. Your head has a tendency to lean to the right or left, and the tilting of one's ear to the side is another indicator that your levator muscles are over-activated.

Muscle tension headaches are also a result of these muscles groups being irritated or inflamed. The common act of placing the phone between your ear and shoulder to support the phone without your hands even for a short period of time can cause a chain reaction in your spine and compensation to occur in your posture, limiting your motion.

CENTERING YOUR HEAD OVER YOUR SHOULDERS

Once you're aware of this head-forward problem, it's fairly easy to correct. Sitting in your car is the best place to correct this problem: first, raise your headrest so that the back of your head is center with it. Next, straighten your chair to the most upright position. Relax your shoulders back against the seat without pressing them back with a muscular effort. Rise up in the seat, lifting your ribcage as you pull in your abdominal muscles. Then while looking straight ahead, tip your chin slightly down while pushing your head back against the headrest and hold this position for five seconds before relaxing and then repeat.

This process lengthens out your spine while realigning your spine and bringing your head center over your body while replacing your body's center of gravity. From a side view your ears should be even with your shoulders. Immediately you will feel the tension come off your traps and levator neck muscles while you may feel the tiny muscles behind your head working to maintain this position.

If you are sitting in a chair at your work or home, simply follow the above directions, except you won't have a headrest, so instead place your index finger against your chin and as you press your chin back your head will follow into position and hold and release as before.

PERFECTING YOUR POSTURE

An ideal posture starts with a strong foundation, creating a balanced structural support that will prevent over developed tight muscles and stiff joints. You are trying to prevent degenerative problems to your major joints down the road now by improving your overall postural flexibility and muscle tone. From a side view your ear is aligned with your shoulder and each arm is resting along your hip and your hip is over your knee, which is over your ankle.

STRETCHING INTO YOUR NEW PERFECT POSTURE

Now we will start at the top of your head and work our way down the body, stretching out your postural muscles to gain more flexibility throughout your body. These exercises are also a good warm-up for the other stretches in the book. Take your time and remember not to force yourself into a position and breathe in a relaxed manner during the duration of your movements.

NECK AND SHOULDERS STRETCHES— WALL STRETCH WITH ARM SWING

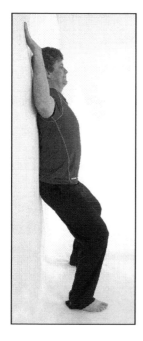 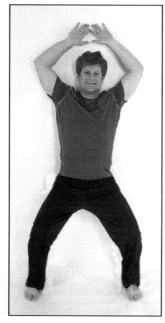

1. Begin by standing with your back against the wall, your feet shoulder width apart and a few feet from the wall. Your knees are bent so your thighs are parallel to the floor.

2. Place your arms up against the wall, bent at the elbows (as if you are holding a crossing-guard sign).

3. With your hands in an open position, keep your wrists, head, and entire back flat against the wall and tuck your chin slightly downward.

4. From this position slowly raise your arms up and toward each other until they come together at the top of your head—hold for three seconds before returning until your arms are parallel to the floor again. Hold and repeat.

Key Points to Remember
- Keep your whole back against the wall during the entire movement

LEVATOR STRETCH

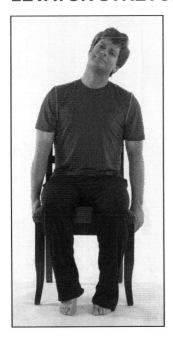

1. Start by sitting in a chair with your knees and feet together and your back supported against the back of the chair. Your head is even over your shoulders and you're looking straight ahead.

2. Place your arms down by your sides and let them hang loose. Next, take your right hand with your arm straight and clasp the side of the chair with your fingers and hold this position.

3. Next, tip your left ear toward your left shoulder, feeling the stretch along the right side of your neck down into the shoulder. Hold the position briefly less than two seconds before returning your head to the neutral position and repeat before switching to your left hand.

KEY POINTS TO REMEMBER:
- Do not do the stretch if you have any type of disc-related injury to your neck region.
- Remember to clasp your hand on the chair, not pull your hand down.

- Remember to not force your head down or away from your neutral position

- You just need a small amount of movement to benefit from the stretch

SHOULDER SQUEEZE

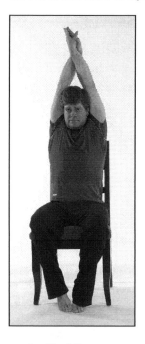

1. Start the movement standing or sitting with your arms down by your sides and relaxed with your head over your shoulder while looking straight ahead. Feet are about shoulder-width apart with a slight bend in your knees.

2. Next raise your arms up and out to the sides of your body and over your head while inhaling.

3. From this position grasp your hands together gently and reach up above your head while squeezing your shoulder blades back and hold at the top position for three seconds before relaxing your hands and lowering your arms down by your sides while exhaling. Repeat the movement.

KEY POINTS TO REMEMBER:

- Remember to reach as high as you can with your arms.

- Don't arch your back during the movement.

SHRUGS

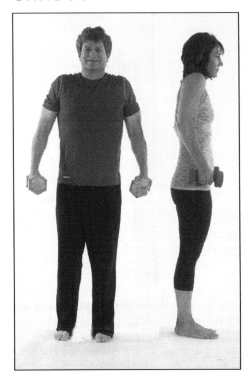

1. Start this movement with your feet shoulder-width apart and your arms relaxed by your sides with your head over your shoulders while looking straight ahead.

2. Next slowly raise your shoulders up toward your ears while inhaling and at the top of the movement begin to roll your shoulders back while squeezing your shoulder blades together.

3. Slowly lower your arms down behind you while exhaling and bring them back to the starting position and repeat.

4. After your warm-up set, grab a pair of light dumbbells and repeat the exercise as before.

KEY POINTS TO REMEMBER:
- Remember to raise your arms up toward your ears as high as you can go.
- Remember to always squeeze your arms back.
- Don't hold your breath while performing the exercise.

SHRUG PRESSES

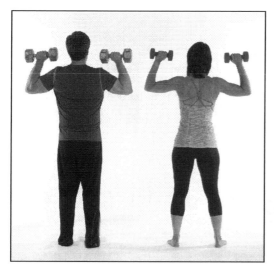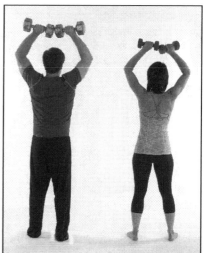

1. Start this movement with your feet shoulder-width apart and holding a pair of dumbbells in your hands with your arms relaxed by your sides with your head aligned over your shoulders while looking straight ahead.

2. Slowly curl the dumbbells up toward your shoulders and slowly rotate your hands so that your palms are facing out as you raise your arms over your head.

3. Begin squeezing your shoulder blades together while exhaling as you press the weights up and over your head to touch the dumbbells at the top of the movement.

4. From the top position inhale as you lower the dumbbells in the same sequence as before until you are in the starting position, and repeat.

KEY POINTS TO REMEMBER:

• Remember to maintain the neutral spine position with your head over your shoulders while looking straight ahead.

• Do not look down during the exercise at any time.

• Remember to squeeze your shoulder blades back while pressing over your head at the same time. Really feel your upper back postural muscles working during the movement.

• Keep your arms back far enough so that when your hands come along they are even with your ears and not in front of your face when pressing over your head.

SEATED SQUATS

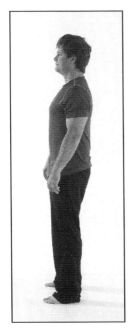 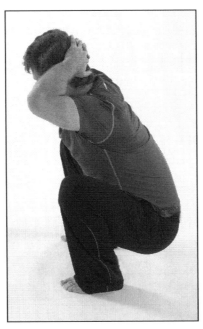

1. Begin with feet shoulder-width apart and arms relaxed by your side. Slowly bend your knees as far as you can go without placing any stress on your knee joints.

2. In this position slowly lower your hips down toward the floor while placing your hands behind your head. A modification of this movement (if you do not have the range of motion yet) is to hold onto a chair or place your hand on a wall for balance. The key is to relax your back and leg muscles in the down position. Hold for three seconds and rise up to the start position and repeat.

KEY POINTS TO REMEMBER:

- Remember to keep your back straight throughout the movement. Don't round your back or shoulders.

- Maintain your heels on the ground or place something underneath your heels at first until you improve your flexibility.

TABLE STRETCH

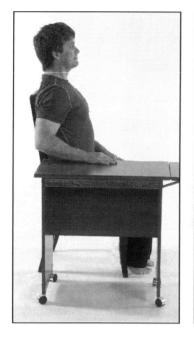 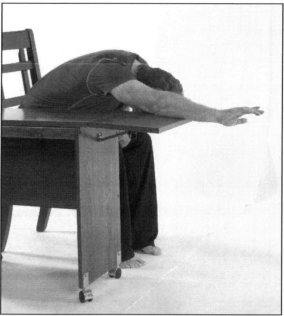

1. Start the movement with your feet slightly wider than shoulder-width apart and your arms down by your sides while you are looking straight ahead in front of a table, counter, or chair.

2. Begin by raising your arms straight out in front of you while bending at your waist only until your hands are resting on the surface with your palms down.

3. From here shift your weight back onto your heels while pressing your hands down and slightly pulling back. Hold the stretch for five to ten seconds before releasing the position and return to the upright standing position.

KEY POINTS TO REMEMBER:

- Remember not to arch or round your back during the exercise.

- Remember to keep your knees slightly bent and not in a locked position during the movement.

- Keep your neck and shoulders relaxed while pulling back.

- Keep your heels down during the exercise at all times.

LYING ON BACK PULLING KNEE ACROSS STRETCH

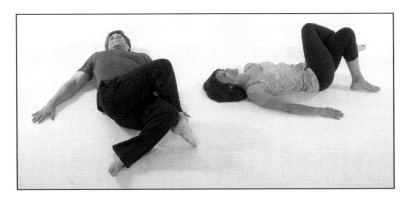

1. Start the exercise by lying on your back, bend knees and relaxed with your arms down by your sides. Keep looking straight with your chin slightly elevated while looking up.

2. Bend your right knee and rest your right foot next to your left knee or higher.

3. Next place your right hand on the right side of your bent knee and slowly press your right thigh across the center of your left leg without lifting your right hip off the floor. Hold for three seconds and return to the start position and repeat before continuing with the opposite leg.

KEY POINTS TO REMEMBER:

- Remember to not twist your leg over your body.

- Remember not to twist your spine during the movement.

- Keep your lower back flat during the exercise.

- Remember to maintain the end position for three seconds to benefit from the exercise.

- Do not force your leg over; instead, relax into the exercise while breathing normally.

CHEST OPENER

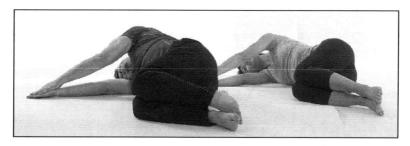

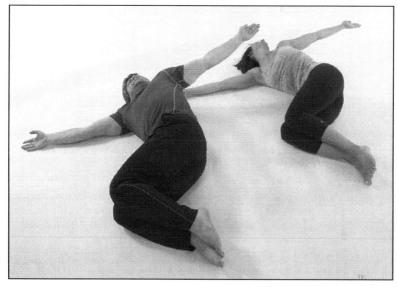

1. Start the exercise by lying on your right side, with your knees bent your arms outstretched and relaxed hands together.

2. Next keeping your left arm straight begin bring your arm up and over while turning your head in the same direction.

3. Try to bring your arm even with your shoulder height throughout the movement. Hold for three seconds and return to the start position and repeat before continuing with the opposite side.

KEY POINTS TO REMEMBER:

• Remember not to twist your spine during the movement.

CHAPTER SUMMARY

- Gravitational forces can take their toll on our joints and spinal alignment.

- Change your posture every twenty minutes.

- Do not let your body become stiff and accustomed to holding onto a particular posture for too long.

- Change the angle of your car seat from the morning to evening to help maintain normal back and neck support.

- Be conscious of your posture while in motion as well as when exercising.

- Avoid an overprotecting posture. Remember that it is important to maintain an overall relaxed posture to avoid restricting movements by clenching muscles and adopting an unnatural, stiff posture.

- Do these postural stretching exercises daily.

- Your new better posture will make you look thinner, more confident and stand taller.

CHAPTER 4

WALL STRETCHES— A PARTNER TO ENHANCE YOUR FLEXIBILITY

This is one training partner you can count on to always be there no matter where you are—your house, office, gym, airport—there will always be a wall for you to stretch on. You can use as little or as much force against the wall without concern of your body weight or fitness level to start these movements. You will be amazed at how many muscle groups you can actively stretch in a short period of time.

These stretches have been career savers for many of my top competitive athletes as well my other patients, they're easy to do and I will share with you in a step-by-step manner how to perform them safely and in the most productive way in this chapter.

WALL TURNS

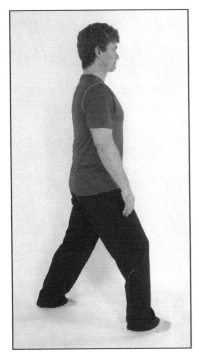 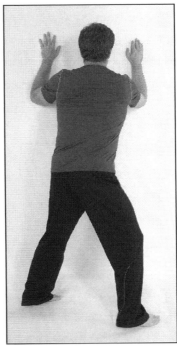

MUSCLE AND JOINT EMPHASIS:
Back, deltoid, obliques, hip flexors, and chest muscles.

THE POSITIONING:
Begin by standing with your legs shoulder width apart with your arms by your sides about a foot away from the wall with your left side facing the wall.

THE MOVEMENT:
1. Step forward with your right foot into a front stance placing 70 percent of your weight onto your right foot. Step back with your left foot making sure your left foot is pointing ahead like your right foot.

2. Turn your upper body so your chest faces the wall and raise your arms at or above shoulder height with a bend in your elbows.

3. Next place your left hand on the wall then your right hand pressing your palms and forearms against the wall.

4. Next lean your upper body into the wall feeling the stretch in your shoulder and back regions. All while maintaining your arm position against the wall at all times. Return to step two position and repeat for the number of repetitions and repeat on the opposite side.

KEY POINTS TO REMEMBER:

- Focus on relaxing into the stretch.

- Keep your arms against the wall for the best stretch possible.

- Do not twist your spine rather gentle turn at your waistline through the range of motion without leaning towards the wall.

- Concentrate on holding your abdominal muscles in during the duration of the exercise.

- Do not force your joint or muscle into the range of motion.

- Maintain an upright posture.

WALL TURNS #2

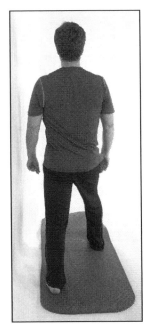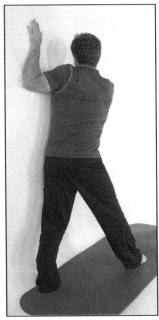

MUSCLE AND JOINT EMPHASIS:

Back, deltoid, obliques, hip flexors, and chest muscles.

THE POSITIONING:

Begin by standing with your legs shoulder width apart with your arms by your sides about a foot away from the wall with your left side facing the wall.

THE MOVEMENT:

1. Step forward with your right foot into a front stance placing 70 percent of your weight onto your right foot. Step back with your left foot making sure your left foot is pointing ahead like your right foot.

2. Turn your upper body so your chest faces the wall and raise your arms at or above shoulder height with a bend in your elbows.

3. Next place your arms outstretched at shoulder height and press your palms and forearms against the wall.

4. Next lean your hips towards the wall feeling the stretch in your shoulder and back regions. All while maintaining your arm position against the wall at all times. Then slowly shift 70 percent of your weight on your back foot. Return to step two position and repeat for the number of repetitions and repeat on the opposite side.

FRONT KICK WALL STRETCH

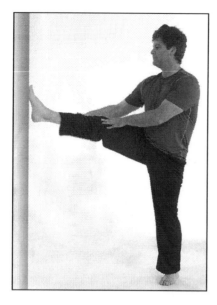

MUSCLE AND JOINT EMPHASIS:
Hamstrings, calves, hip flexors, glutes and lower back.

THE POSITIONING:
Begin by standing with your legs shoulder width apart with your arms by your sides about three feet away from the wall.

THE MOVEMENT:

1. Bend your right knee up toward your chest and hold your leg with your hands around your knee region while maintaining your balance.

2. Next extend your right leg out toward the wall until your foot is touching the wall at least waist high to shoulder height. Place your hands along your right leg either at the knee joint or lower calf while bending at the waist maintaining your balance.

3. Hold this outstretched position for three to five seconds before returning to the bent knee position and then repeat without touching your foot to the floor for a set of repetitions and then repeat with the opposite leg.

KEY POINTS TO REMEMBER:

- Focus on relaxing into the stretch.

- Keep your leg up as high as you can against the wall for the best stretch possible.

- Do not hunch over your leg rather lean at your waist while maintaining an upright posture.

- Concentrate on holding your abdominal muscles in during the duration of the exercise.

- Do not force your joint or muscle into the range of motion.

- You can place a chair next to you at first to help with balance and help you hold the stretch longer.

FRONT KICK AND FLOOR TOUCH WALL STRETCH

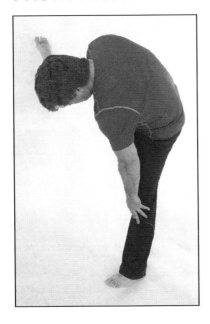

MUSCLE AND JOINT EMPHASIS:
Hamstrings, calves, hip flexors, glutes and lower back.

THE POSITIONING:
Begin by standing with your legs shoulder width apart with your arms by your sides about three feet away from the wall.

THE MOVEMENT:

1. Bend your right knee up toward your chest and hold your leg with your hands around your knee region while maintaining your balance.

2. Next extend your right leg out toward the wall until your foot is touching the wall at least waist high to shoulder height. Place your hands along your right leg either at the knee joint or lower calf while bending at the waist maintaining your balance.

3. Then Take your left arm and drop it down towards the floor along your left leg. If you can hold onto your ankle or touch the floor with your hand for a deeper stretch.

4. Hold this stretch position for three to five seconds before returning to the bent knee position and then repeat without touching your foot to the floor for a set of repetitions and then repeat with the opposite leg.

KEY POINTS TO REMEMBER:

- Focus on relaxing into the stretch.

- Keep your leg up as high as you can against the wall for the best stretch possible.

- Concentrate on holding your abdominal muscles in during the duration of the exercise.

SIDE KICK WALL STRETCH

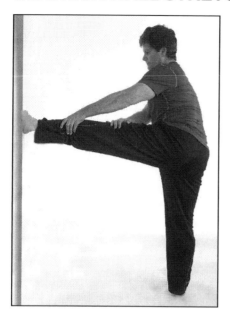

MUSCLE AND JOINT EMPHASIS:

Hamstrings, adductors, abductors, glutes, calves, hip flexors and lower back.

THE POSITIONING:

Begin by standing with your legs shoulder width apart with your arms by your sides about three feet away from the wall. Next turn your left side toward the wall.

THE MOVEMENT:

1. Bend your left knee up toward your side, chest height and hold your leg with your hands around your knee region while maintaining your balance.

2. Next extend your left leg out toward the wall until your foot is touching the wall at least waist high to shoulder height. Place your hands along your right leg either at the knee joint or lower calf while bending at the waist maintaining your balance.

3. Hold this outstretched position for three to five seconds before returning to the bent knee position and then repeat without touching your foot to the floor for a set of repetitions and then repeat with the opposite leg.

KEY POINTS TO REMEMBER:

• Keep your leg up as high as you can against the wall for the best stretch possible.

• Do not hunch over your leg rather lean at your waist while maintaining an upright posture.

• Concentrate on holding your abdominal muscles in during the duration of the exercise.

• You can place a chair next to you at first to help with balance and help you hold the stretch longer.

SIDE KICK WALL STRETCH AND
FLOOR TOUCH WALL STRETCH

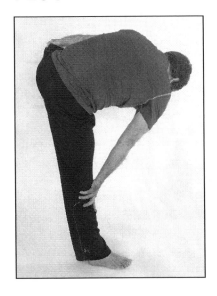

MUSCLE AND JOINT EMPHASIS:
Hamstrings, adductors, abductors, glutes, calves, hip flexors and lower back.

THE POSITIONING:
Begin by standing with your legs shoulder width apart with your arms by your sides about three feet away from the wall. Next turn your left side toward the wall.

THE MOVEMENT:

1. Bend your left knee up toward your side, chest height and hold your leg with your hands around your knee region while maintaining your balance.

2. Next extend your left leg out toward the wall until your foot is touching the wall at least waist high to shoulder height. Place your hands along your left leg either at the knee joint or lower calf while bending at the waist maintaining your balance.

3. Hold this outstretched position for three to five seconds, then reach down with your right arm along your right leg reaching toward the floor, before returning to the bent knee position and then repeat without touching your foot to the floor for a set of repetitions and then repeat with the opposite leg.

KEY POINTS TO REMEMBER:

• Keep your leg up as high as you can against the wall for the best stretch possible.

• Do not hunch over your leg rather lean at your waist while maintaining an upright posture.

• Concentrate on holding your abdominal muscles in during the duration of the exercise.

• You can place a chair next to you at first to help with balance and help you hold the stretch longer.

HAMSTRING STRETCH AWAY FROM THE WALL

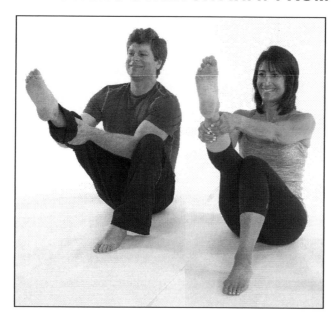

MUSCLE AND JOINT EMPHASIS:
Hamstrings, adductors, abductors, glutes, calves, hip flexors and lower back.

THE POSITIONING:
Begin by sitting with your legs shoulder width apart and your arms by your sides, your back and shoulder blades against the wall.

THE MOVEMENT:

1. Bend your knees keeping your feet flat on the floor and your arms by your sides.

2. Next extend your right leg straight with a slightly bend in the knee keeping your back against the wall guide your leg with your hands and slightly pull your leg toward your head gently. Hold the end position for three to five seconds before returning to the start position and repeat for the number of repetitions and repeat with the opposite leg. .

KEY POINTS TO REMEMBER:

- Focus on relaxing into the stretch.

- Keep your shoulder blades back against the wall for the best stretch possible.

- Do not pull back hard on your leg rather gentle guide your leg through the range of motion without pulling away from the wall.

- Concentrate on holding your abdominal muscles in during the duration of the exercise.

PIRIFORMIS STRETCH AWAY FROM THE WALL

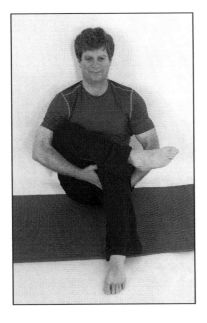

MUSCLE AND JOINT EMPHASIS:
Hamstrings, adductors, abductors, glutes, calves, hip flexors and lower back.

THE POSITIONING:
Begin by seating with your legs shoulder width apart with your arms by your sides and your back and shoulder blades against the wall.

THE MOVEMENT:

1. Bend your knees keeping your feet flat on the floor and your arms by your sides.

2. Next bend your right leg at the knee and place your right ankle resting on your left knee.

3. Then guide your right leg up with your hands behind your left knee slightly pull your leg toward your chest gently. Hold the end position for three to five seconds before returning to the start position and repeat for the number of repetitions and repeat with the opposite leg for a set.

KEY POINTS TO REMEMBER:

- Focus on relaxing into the stretch.

- Concentrate on pulling in you abdominal muscles during the duration of the exercise.

- Keep your shoulder blades back against the wall for the best stretch possible.

- Do not pull back hard on your legs rather gentle guide your leg through the range of motion without pulling away from the wall

SEATED LEG SPLITS AWAY FROM THE WALL

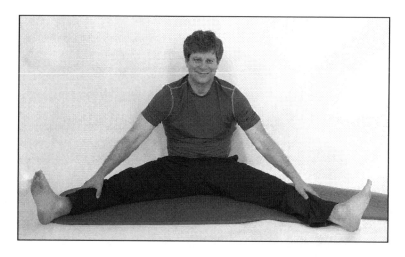

MUSCLE AND JOINT EMPHASIS:
hips, hamstrings, piriformis, glutes, and lower back muscles

THE POSITIONING:
Begin by sitting on the floor with your legs out stretched to the side and your arms by your sides with your back against the wall.

THE MOVEMENT:
1. Begin by sitting on the floor with your legs out stretched to the side and your arms by your sides with your back against the wall.

2. Next bending at the waist and lean forward and hold this new position again before returning to the upright position with your arms by your side then repeat on the opposite side and repeat alternating between sides for a complete set.

KEY POINTS TO REMEMBER
- Do not round your back when performing this movement.
- Relax and breathe deeply during the stretch.
- Maintain a steady rhythm in your speed during the exercise.

STANDING PIRIFORMIS WALL STRETCH

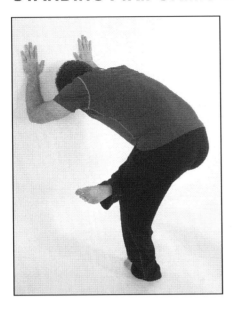

MUSCLE AND JOINT EMPHASIS:
Muscles emphases: hip joint, piriformis, abductors, adductors, TFL band, hamstrings and lower back muscles

THE POSITIONING:
Begin by standing with your legs shoulder width apart with your arms by your sides about a foot from the wall.

THE MOVEMENT:

1. Bend your right knee and turn your leg across toward your left leg resting above the knee higher while placing your right hand against the wall for support. Use your left hand to help raise and pull your right knee across your body.

2. Next lean forward with your upper body towards the wall resting against the wall with your upper body if you can and hold this position for three to five seconds before lowering your leg and switching legs and alternating in between repetitions.

KEY POINTS TO REMEMBER

- Focus on relaxing into the stretch.

- Concentrate on pulling in you abdominal muscles during the duration of the exercise.

- Do not force your joint or muscle into the range of motion.

- Keep your leg raise as high as possible for the best stretch possible.

- Do not pull back hard on your leg rather gentle guide your leg through the range of motion.

FROGGIE STRETCH ON THE WALL

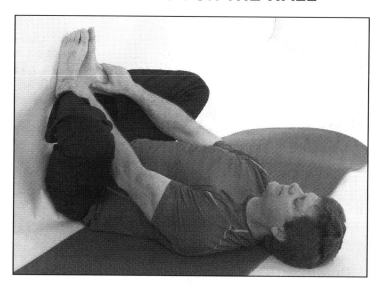

MUSCLE AND JOINT EMPHASIS:
Hamstrings, adductors, abductors, glutes, calves, hip flexors and lower back.

THE POSITIONING:
Begin by lying on your back with your hips up against the wall as close as possible and your feet resting on the wall with your legs outstretched with your arms down by your side.

THE MOVEMENT:

1. Bend your knees keeping the bottom of your feet together and against the wall.

2. Next slide your feet down as you drop your knees off to the sides trying to bring them touching the floor. Place your hands on your feet to further lower your legs into position and hold for three to five seconds before extending your legs straight to the top of the wall and repeat for the number of repetitions.

KEY POINTS TO REMEMBER:

• Keep your hips against the wall for the best stretch possible.

• Do not pull back hard on your feet rather gentle guide your legs through the range of motion without pulling away from the wall.

• Concentrate on holding your abdominal muscles in during the duration of the exercise.

• Keep the bottom of your feet together at all times to activate the inner and outer leg muscles.

HURDLERS STRETCH ON THE WALL

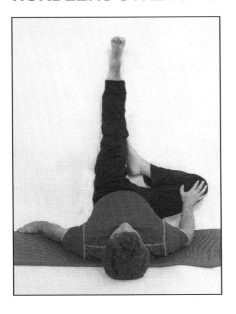

MUSCLE AND JOINT EMPHASIS:
Hamstrings, adductors, abductors, glutes, calves, hip flexors and lower back.

THE POSITIONING:
Begin by lying on your back with your hips up against the wall as close as possible and your feet resting on the wall with your legs outstretched with your arms down by your side resting on the floor.

THE MOVEMENT:

1. Bend your right knee keeping the bottom of your foot against your left leg against the wall.

2. Next use your right hand and press your right knee down toward the wall while pulling your left toes back, flexing your left foot and hold this position for three to five seconds before extending your legs straight to the top of the wall and repeat for the number of repetitions before switching to the opposite leg.

KEY POINTS TO REMEMBER:

• Keep your hips against the wall for the best stretch possible.

• Do not push hard on your knee joint rather lean your hand onto your thigh through the range of motion along the wall.

• Concentrate on holding your abdominal muscles in during the duration of the exercise.

• Do not arch your lower back off the floor during the movement

HURDLERS REACH STRETCH ON THE WALL

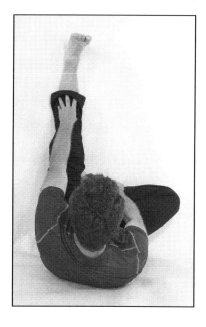

MUSCLE AND JOINT EMPHASIS:
Hamstrings, adductors, abductors, glutes, calves, hip flexors and lower back.

THE POSITIONING:
Begin by lying on your back with your hips up against the wall as close as possible and your feet resting on the wall with your legs outstretched with your arms down by your side resting on the floor.

THE MOVEMENT:

1. Bend your right knee keeping the bottom of your foot against your left leg against the wall.

2. Next use your right hand and press your right knee down toward the wall while pulling your left toes back, flexing your left foot while reaching up with your left hand and hold this position for three to five seconds before extending your legs straight to the top of the wall and repeat for the number of repetitions before switching to the opposite leg.

KEY POINTS TO REMEMBER:

• Do not over reach with your extended arm.

• Keep your hips against the wall for the best stretch possible.

• Do not push hard on your knee joint rather lean your hand onto your thigh through the range of motion along the wall.

• Do not arch your lower back off the floor during the movement

CHAPTER 5

TOWEL STRETCHES—
HEALING MOVES: HOW TO RELIEVE
AND PREVENT STIFFNESS GENTLY

This chapter was written after many people came up to me after one of my *BackSmart* stretching seminars and told me how they enjoyed the session and how could they do more to improve upon what they have just learn. Some of them have been going to some type of yoga class before coming to my seminar and a few achieved greater flexibility from doing the yoga while others spoke of disappointment in not getting faster results. They wanted to spend less time performing the different poses because they felt frustrated or limited. While not knowing who had taught them before, I could only tell them that it takes time to improve upon their flexibility and that yoga is an art form and there are many levels to it and if they did not have the patience or time they could use the *Basksmart* Daily Dozen and the towel stretches to accelerate their goals. Like the ladder I mention in the *BackSmart Fitness Plan*, there are many things available to enhance your flexibility with some use of your imagination.

BENEFITS

The towel is carried around with most people who work out or is readily available to them to use. A common phrase often heard is "If only I was just a little bit taller or just a little bit thinner my life would be much easier? While this chapter doesn't promise you new height or that you will become a lot thinner it will help you improve your flexibility in a low-impact way while being highly effective at the same time. By extending your ability to reach a tad farther or place your body in a position once before was not an attainable not only will you become stronger and more flexible with your new found range of motion you will have further prevented future injuries from occurring from stiff and inflexible muscles and joints in a safe, control manner.

I have worked the towel stretches into many of my patients and athletes' routine when they were out on the golf course, tennis or basketball court and there was no dry or soft ground to do the *BackSmart* Daily Dozen stretches. These stretches are highly effective exercises that will build flexibility while strengthening apposing muscle groups by just using a towel and a small area of space. I recommend these movements to be performed before your exercise program, especially for sports that require using a club or a racket or any type of throwing or shooting motion. Follow up these stretches with the *BackSmart* Daily Dozen when you have completed your activity.

If you are the type of person who is very inflexible you will enjoy using the towel stretches because you will gain greater range of motion in a shorter period of time by extending your fulcrum point away from your body causing a deeper stretch to occur in your muscles thus enhancing your flexibility. Performing these stretches will reduce the likelihood of injuries and increase your power and flexibility in your arms and legs that are common sites of injuries for most athletic people besides the spinal region.

The Towel stretches can be done at any level of flexibility, and people at all levels should complete each stretch as follows: 2 to 4 total sets of 10 to 12 repetitions, holding each stretch for 30 seconds to a minute. As you become more familiar with the movements, you can repeat the sequence as often as you would like to further enhance your flexibility.

TOWEL PULL

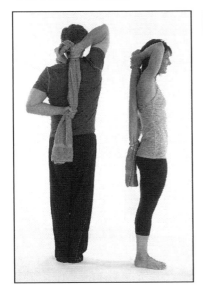 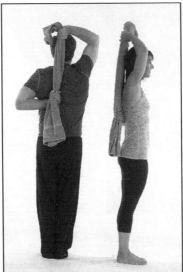

This stretch will improve your flexibility in your shoulder and back muscles while increasing your gripping strengthen in the process. This movement will stretch your muscles at a different angle thus improving your range of motion and enhancing your athletic ability while preventing injuries to these important postural muscle groups. Great stretch to do before throwing a ball, tennis or swimming to give you that extra edge.

THE MOVEMENT:
1. Start By holding your right arm overhead holding the towel then bend your elbow and drop your hand down behind your head.

2. Place your left hand behind your back and hold the towel taunt.

3. Begin pulling up with your right hand allowing your left arm with bent elbow to glide up and hold.

4. Next lower back down and slightly pull downward and hold. Repeat for set of repetitions before switching arm positions.

KEY POINTS TO REMEMBER:
- Focus on relaxing into the stretch.
- Keep looking straight ahead maintaining good posture.
- Concentrate on holding your abdominal muscles in during the duration of the exercise.
- Do not force your joint or muscle into the range of motion.

TOWEL CIRCLES

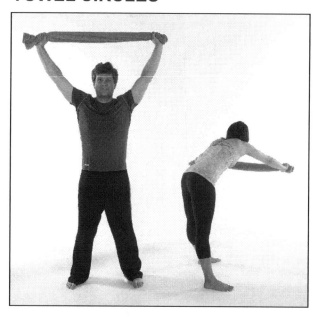

Great movement to loosen up your waistline as well as your shoulders. Maintain good posture when performing this movement.

THE MOVEMENT:

1. Start with your arms over head with the towel between your hands.

2. Pull your hands out to the side keeping your arms above your head. Then reach up as far as you can with your hands maintaining the tension on the towel.

3. Next bend at the waist keeping your stomach muscles pulled in bend forward until your upper body is parallel to the floor.

4. Begin rotating your upper body maintaining your arms out stretched the duration of the movement.

5. Start counter clockwise then reverse direction for set of repetitions return to the upright position and repeat clockwise.

KEY POINTS TO REMEMBER:

• Focus on relaxing into the stretch.

• Exhale, don't hold your breath while performing the movement

• Concentrate on holding your abdominal muscles in during the duration of the exercise.

BENT OVER SHOULDER/ TRICEPS STRETCH

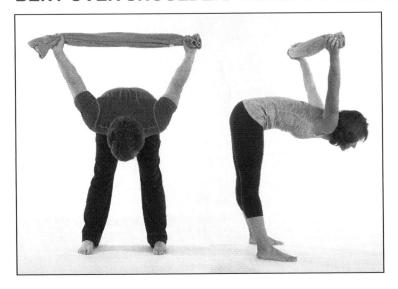

Start with your feet shoulder width apart holding the towel with both hands behind your back at waist level. Arms are straight.

THE MOVEMENT:

1. Begin by pulling your hands out to the side keeping the tension constant during the movement.

2. Bend at the waist as you raise your arms up toward the ceiling moving them forward above your head.

3. Hold for ten seconds before returning to the start position and repeat.

Don't do the movement if you have any shoulder pain or discomfort.

KEY POINTS TO REMEMBER:

- Focus on relaxing into the stretch.

- Maintain a neutral head position while performing the movement

- Do not force your joint or muscle into the range of motion.

TRICEPS STRETCH

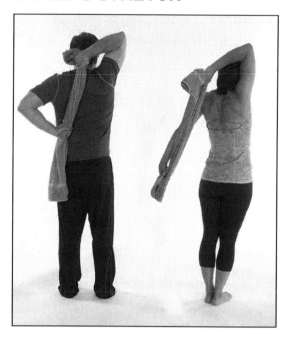

THE MOVEMENT:

1. Start By holding your right arm overhead holding the towel.

2. Bend your elbow and drop your hand down behind your head.

3. Begin pulling up with your right hand while pulling your left arm out to the side of your body straighten your left arm and hold the position for ten seconds.

4. Repeat for set of repetitions before switching arm positions.

KEY POINTS TO REMEMBER:

• Keep looking straight ahead maintaining good posture.

• Concentrate on holding your abdominal muscles in during the duration of the exercise.

• Do not force your joint or muscle into the range of motion.

DOOR OR PARTNER STRETCH

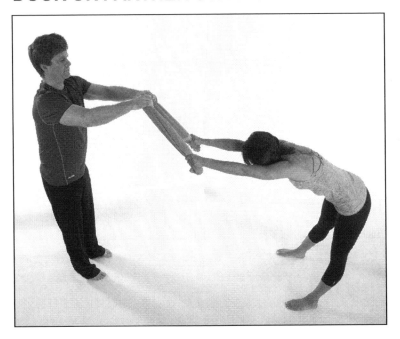

This stretch will improve your overall flexibility in your shoulder and upper back and neck regions while increasing your gripping strengthen in the process. This movement will stretch your muscles at a different angle thus improving your range of motion and enhancing your athletic ability while preventing injuries to these important postural muscle groups. Great stretch to do before biking, swimming or golf to give you that extra edge.

THE MOVEMENT:

1. Start by placing the towel around a pole, chin up bar or above a door. Sturdy enough to support your body weight when you lean back. Stand at the length of the towel while holding on with both hands.

2. Bend your knees slightly and bend at your waist while pulling back with your hands and hold 30 seconds to 1 minute then relax to a standing position then repeat the movement.

KEY POINTS TO REMEMBER

- Maintain a neutral head position during the movement.

- Concentrate on holding your abdominal muscles in during the duration of the exercise.

HURDLE STRETCH WITH TOWEL

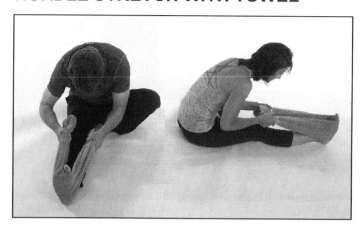

Now that we have worked the upper body and shoulder region it is time to concentrate on the lower half of the body. Lower body stretching is very important in improving your stamina and longevity in your chosen sport activities. Once people develop injuries to their lower body they develop gate changes and limits their range of motion and athletic potential. Don't let this happen to you, focus on the muscles being stretched and you will see improvements quickly.

This stretch will increase your upper and lower leg regions and lower back flexibility enhancing your range of motion for faster speed and endurance activities.

THE MOVEMENT:

1. Start by sitting down on the floor with your right leg in front of you with your left foot tucked in by your right leg.

2. Place the towel over your right foot holding onto it with both hands.

3. Slowly bend forward with your upper body while pulling back on the towel. Breathe deeply and relax into the stretch holding this position for 30 seconds to a minute.

4. Repeat for set of repetitions before stretching legs.

KEY POINTS TO REMEMBER:

- Focus on relaxing into the stretch.

- Relax your upper body while maintaining good posture.

- Concentrate on holding your abdominal muscles in during the duration of the exercise.

- Do not force your joint or muscle into the range of motion.

SPLITS WITH A TOWEL

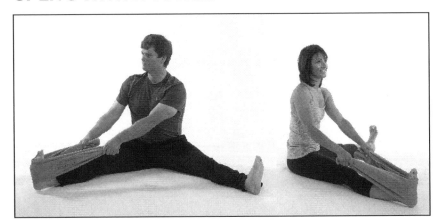

A very effective stretch that will increase your flexibility in regions of the inner and back of the thigh areas that are commonly injured during sporting activities. This movement will increase your motion in these often-difficult muscle groups to isolate a true stretch from.

THE MOVEMENT:

1. Start by sitting on the floor with your legs apart.

2. Place the towel over your right foot while holding on with both hands.

3. Slowly lower your upper body while pulling your arms towards you. Hold for 30 seconds to 1 minute and repeat on the opposite side alternating between repetitions.

KEY POINTS TO REMEMBER:

- Focus on relaxing into the stretch.

- Keep looking straight ahead maintaining good posture.

- Concentrate on holding your abdominal muscles in during the duration of the exercise.

HAMSTRING STRETCH

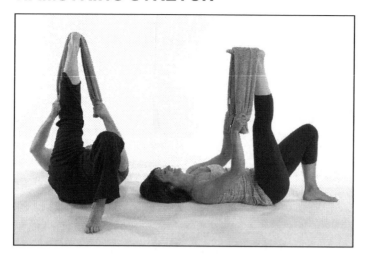

This movement emphasizes the back of the upper and lower legs muscles and the hip flexors group, which are commonly tight among most of the population which can slow you down during your activities and tight hamstring muscles can set you up for many leg and lower back injuries.

THE MOVEMENT:

1. Start by lying on your back and raise your right leg upwards to 90 degrees from the floor with the towel resting over the foot.

2. Holding the towel with both hands pull the leg back toward your head. Relax and breathe deeply while holding the end position for a two count. Then repeat on the opposite side alternating between repetitions.

KEY POINTS TO REMEMBER

• Keep your head down on the floor.

• Concentrate on holding your abdominal muscles in during the duration of the exercise.

PIRIFORMIS STRETCH

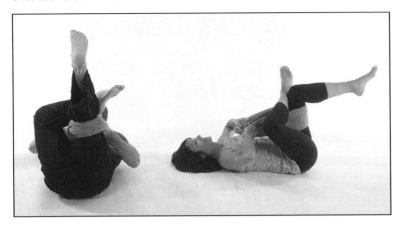

This stretch relaxes one of the tightest muscles in the body that causes Many problems from sciatica (leg pain) to limiting hip rotating and lunging which are all important movements to enhance your endurance and athletic ability.

THE MOVEMENT:

1. Start by lying on your back. Bend your knees and place your feet flat on the ground.

2. Lift your right leg and place your right ankle onto the left leg with the knee bent just above the left knee.

3. Place the towel behind your left knee joint.

4. Holding on with both hands then slowly pull the left leg up towards your left shoulder. You will feel the stretch in the right leg down by the buttocks and hamstrings.

5. Then pulls towards your right shoulder slightly bring your legs across your body. This movement will stretch the muscle group from a different angle. Complete one set of repetitions on one side then repeat with the other leg.

Reminder: Many people perform this stretch incorrectly by just bending the legs toward their chest rather then up to the shoulder area, this will limit your flexibility and may set you up for injuries when running, biking or climbing.

KEY POINTS TO REMEMBER

- Focus stretching your lower body.

- Keep your head down on the floor.

- Do not over pull with your arms to bring your leg up.

CHAPTER SUMMARY

- By using something as practical as a towel you can enhance your flexibility safely and effectively without comprising your muscles or joints in the process.

- You are able to achieve greater range of motion without forcing your body into any uncomfortable positions or contortions to achieve your goals nor do you have to be born flexible.

- Use the stretches in conjunction with the *BackSmart* Daily Dozen Stretches will execrate your progress and improve your shape and define your body parts with these exercises when performed daily.

- These individual exercise can be combined in different orders and personalized during your training rest periods to speed up your recovery period and further improve your ultimate goal of a better physic and improved endurance.

- Slow steady movements are important to follow when performing any of these stretches and exercises throughout the book.

- Focus on the muscles you are stretching, do not become distracted or too relaxed when performing the movements.

- Maintain proper body alignment when moving through the exercises and preserve your muscle control while relaxing the other body parts that you are not stretching at that moment in time.

CHAPTER 6

CHAIR AND BALL STRETCHES: RELEASE NERVOUS TENSION

SITTING ON THE BALL

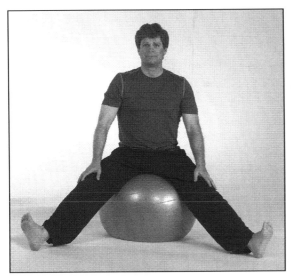

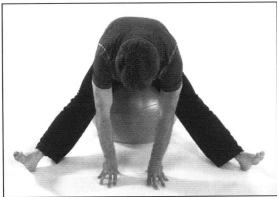

A very effective stretch that will increase your flexibility in regions of your back and hamstrings when you are too stiff to stretch on the floor. This movement will increase your range motion using gravity making it easier to stretch these muscles.

THE MOVEMENT:

1. Start by sitting on the ball with your legs comfortably apart. Your knees are straight.

2. Bend at the waist while reaching forward toward the floor.

3. Hold for 30 seconds to 1 minute, if you can touch the floor great. If not there's a goal for you.

4. Seat back up and repeat moving your legs slightly a part each repetition.

KEY POINTS TO REMEMBER

- Focus on relaxing into the stretch.

- Concentrate on holding your abdominal muscles in during the duration of the exercise.

- Bend at your waist downward rather than leaning forward at the beginning of the movement.

- Breathe and relax into the position.

- **Beginner's cheat** – Bend your knees during the first set and gradually straighten your legs more each time you practice the movement.

MODIFIED HURDLER STRETCH

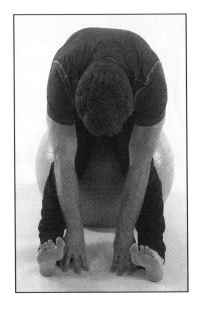

Again another movement that will increase your flexibility in your back,hamstrings, hip flexors, and quads when you are too stiff to stretch on the floor. This movement will increase your range motion using gravity making it easier to stretch these muscles.

THE MOVEMENT:

1. Start by sitting on the ball with your legs comfortably apart. Keep your legs outstretched in front.

2. Bend at the waist while reaching out with your hands toward you're the floor and hold.

3. Hold for 30 seconds to 1 minute, if you can touch the floor If not there's a goal for you.

4. Seat back up and repeat number of repetitions before switching legs.

KEY POINTS TO REMEMBER:

- Focus on relaxing into the stretch.

- Concentrate on holding your abdominal muscles in during the duration of the exercise.

- Bend at your waist downward rather than leaning forward at the beginning of the movement.

- Breathe and relax into the position.

- Don't lean to one side more than the other when bending forward. Try to stay straight as possible.

- **Beginner's cheat –** Bend your knees during the first set and gradually straighten your legs more each time you practice the movement.

BEND OVER STRETCH ON THE BALL

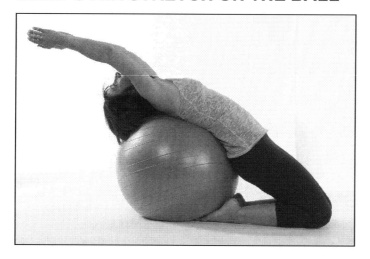

There are unlimited ways of performing this movement based on your level of flexibility. Take your time and you will be rewarded with sweet relief from back stiffness.

THE MOVEMENT:

1. Start by kneeing in front on the ball with your legs comfortably apart or together.

2. Bend backwards over the ball raising your arms over head and back.

3. Reach back while resting your head on the ball until you feel a stretch and hold this position. Hold for 30 seconds to 1 minute.

4. Roll forward until you come back to the beginning at repeat.

KEY POINTS TO REMEMBER:

• Don't start in the kneeling position if you have any knee pains or problems in your knee area.

• **Beginner's cheat** – squat in front of the ball instead of kneeling. Emphases sitting deep before leaning back into the stretch.

• Don't over arch your back instead relax into the position and rest onto the ball.

• **Beginner's cheat**- Place the ball against the wall if you are too stiff to lie onto the ball from the seating position at first.

• Concentrate on holding your abdominal muscles in during the duration of the exercise.

• Breathe and relax into the position.

SIDE LEG STRETCH ON THE BALL

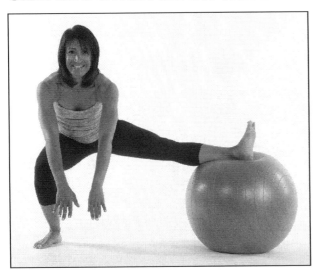

If you never were able to do the splits on the floor when you were younger and wondered how others could do it. Envy no more, this stretch not only stretches your inner and outer leg muscles, it provides core strength and balance as well. Better than the splits!

THE MOVEMENT:
1. Start by squatting on the side of the ball with your legs comfortably apart.

2. Bend your closest knee to the ball while lifting your leg up and over the ball. Straighten your leg as best as possible, while supporting yourself with your hands out stretched on the floor in front of you.

3. Begin slowly to move the leg on the ball away from your body while feeling the stretch in your inner thigh muscles. Hold for 30 seconds to 1 minute.

4. Roll your leg in until you come back to the beginning and repeat before switching legs.

KEY POINTS TO REMEMBER:
- Don't start in the squat position if you have any knee pains or problems in your knee area. Instead start from a standing position.

- **Beginner's cheat** – seat on a chair next to the ball while standing instead.

- Concentrate on holding your abdominal muscles in during the duration of the exercise.

- Breathe and relax into the position.

LYING ON TOP LEG STRETCH ON THE BALL

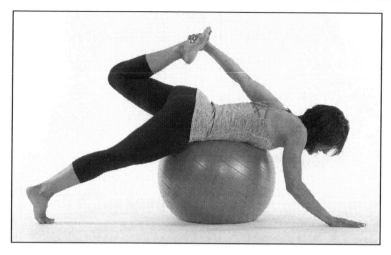

One aspect of using the ball is it is comfortable to get into positions and rest on the ball rather than the a hard surface to be able to gain greater range of motion.

THE MOVEMENT:

1. Start by standing in front on the ball with your legs comfortably apart.

2. Roll onto the ball and place your lower chest or upper stomach on the ball based on your comfort and place your hands on the floor with your arms straight in a push-up position.

3. Your feet are on the floor and your legs are straight.

4. Reach back with your right hand while bending your right knee so you can grab hold of your ankle. Now slowly roll forward and feel the stretch in the top of your thigh and gluteal muscles. Hold for 30 seconds to 1 minute until you come back to the beginning at repeat before switching legs.

5. More advance movement is to raise your foot up toward the ceiling as you lean forward over the ball this will increase the stretch in your hip flexor muscle groups.

KEY POINTS TO REMEMBER:

- Don't bend your knee too hard or hold your ankle if you have any knee pains or problems in your knee area.

- **Beginner's cheat** – If you are unable to hold your ankle start the movement by just bending your knee and try to raise your leg up away from the ball in the stretch position. As you gradually gain flexibility you can try to touch or hold your foot before the ankle.

- Don't over arch your back.

- Concentrate on holding your abdominal muscles in during the duration of the exercise.

- Breathe and relax into the position.

CHAIR STRETCHES: RELEASE NERVOUS TENSION

When you sit for long periods of time your spine tends to compress and your body slips into poor posture; gravity accentuates this problem, as we discussed in chapter three. This can lead to back and neck pain and stiff leg muscles as well. Be it after a long airline flight or sitting and waiting for a few hours, your body is going to tighten up. This prolonged inactivity makes moving more difficult or even painful when you try to stand up. This can occur even while you're sitting at work. No matter how sound your ergonomics chair is your body will suffer from long periods of sitting and inactivity.

This chapter will teach you just how easy it is to complete a full body stretching routine at your chair and even incorporate it into your regular workouts as well. By using different positions, you will be able to stretch out your muscles in a short period of time to remain supple throughout the day.

CHAIR ROTATION STRETCH

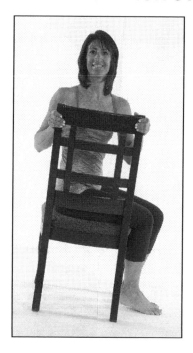

THE MOVEMENT:

1. Start by sitting sideways on a chair with your right hip facing the chair back and your feet on the floor.

2. Place your hands on the chair back as you inhale and sit tall relaxing your upper body.

3. Exhale and rotate your upper body further toward the right and hold the position for 30 seconds before returning to start position

KEY POINTS TO REMEMBER:

- Don't twist your spine or over torque using upper body strength during the movement.

- Relax slowly into positions.

- Allow the chair to aide you into the positions taking weight off your spine and joints.

- Concentrate on holding your abdominal muscles in during the duration of the exercise.

- Breathe deeply.

MID TO UPPER OPEN BACK STRETCH

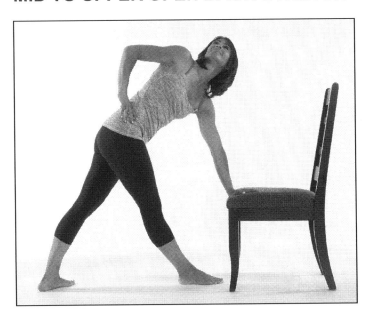

THE MOVEMENT:

1. Begin by placing a chair in front of you and place your right foot forward in a lung position keeping your knee straight.

2. Step back with your left foot maintain your heel flat on the floor and knee is straight.

3. Next place your left hand on the chair and your hand on your right hip.

4. Begin to turn your upper body toward the right and look up over your right shoulder toward the ceiling. Hold this position for 30 seconds before retuning your right arm forward still on your hip and looking straight. Then repeat for repetitions before switching sides.

KEY POINTS TO REMEMBER:

- Don't twist your spine or over torque using upper body strength during the movement.

- Relax slowly into positions.

- Allow the chair to aide you into the positions taking weight off your spine and joints.

- Concentrate on holding your abdominal muscles in during the duration of the exercise.

- Breathe deeply.

MID TO LOWER BACK AND HIP STRETCH

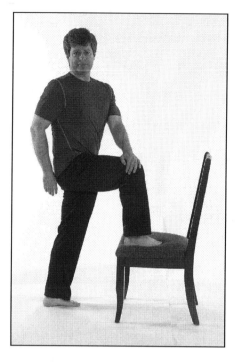

THE MOVEMENT:

1. Standing with feet shoulder width apart, place your right foot on the chair.

2. Next place your left hand on your right knee.

3. Keeping your back straight turn your head towards the right while gently pulling your left hand while bracing with your right leg

4. Hold the position for 30 seconds before returning your hand to the side of your body then repeat for sets of repetitions before switching sides.

KEY POINTS TO REMEMBER:

- Don't twist your spine or over torque using upper body strength during the movement.

- Relax slowly into positions.

- Concentrate on holding your abdominal muscles in during the duration of the exercise.

- Breathe deeply.

LOWER BACK AND HAMSTRING STRETCHES

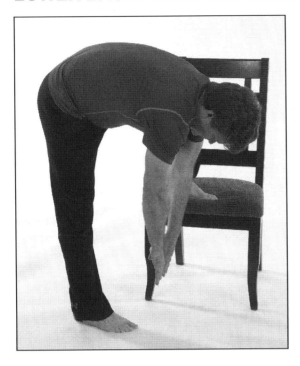

THE MOVEMENT:

1. Standing with feet shoulder width apart with a chair slightly ahead of you off to the left.

2. Place your left foot on the chair.

3. Next reach with your hands down toward the floor.

4. Hold the position for 30 seconds before returning to the upright position then repeat for sets of repetitions before switching sides.

KEY POINTS TO REMEMBER:

• Avoid leaning away from the chair when bending at the waist.

• Relax slowly into the position.

• Allow the chair to aide you into the positions taking weight off your spine and joints.

• Concentrate on holding your abdominal muscles in during the duration of the exercise.

• Breathe deeply.

LOWER BACK HAMSTRING STRETCH NO 2

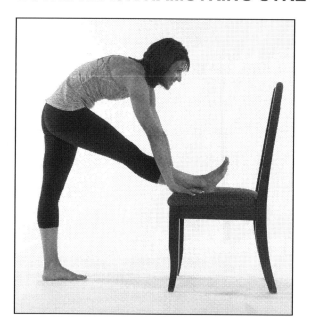

THE MOVEMENT:

1. Stand with your feet shoulder width apart with the chair in front of you about two feet away.

2. Next place your right foot on the chair with your toes pointing up.

3. Then bending at your waist, place your hands on the chair next to your ankle or the bottom of your foot keeping your knees straight throughout the movement.

4. Hold the position for 30 seconds before returning to the upright position then repeat for sets of repetitions before switching sides.

KEY POINTS TO REMEMBER:

- Avoid contracting your hamstrings (back of your leg muscles) during the movement.

- Relax slowly into positions.

- Concentrate on holding your abdominal muscles in during the duration of the exercise.

LOWER MID-BACK AND HAMSTRING STRETCH

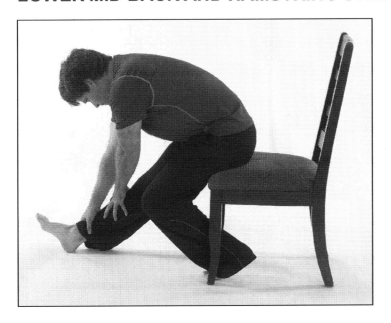

THE MOVEMENT:

1. Sitting upright on a chair with your feet shoulder width apart looking straight ahead.

2. Straighten your right leg out in front of you while bending your left knee so your foot goes under the chair.

3. Next lean forward guiding your upper body down toward your foot with your arms.

4. Hold your hands either at your calf or ankle level, holding for 30 seconds before returning to the upright position then repeat for sets of repetitions before switching sides.

KEY POINTS TO REMEMBER:

- Don't bend your knee

- Relax slowly into positions.

- Allow the chair to aide you into the positions taking weight off your spine and joints.

- Concentrate on holding your abdominal muscles in during the duration of the exercise.

PIRIFORMIS, HIP AND LOWER BACK STRETCH

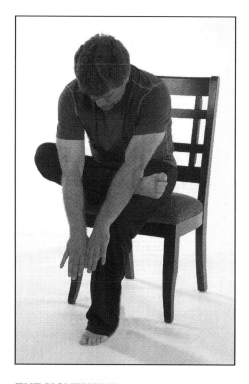

THE MOVEMENT:

1. Sitting upright on a chair with your feet shoulder width apart looking straight ahead.

2. Bending your right leg place your foot on top of your left thigh keeping your left leg.

3. Next lean forward with your upper body down toward your left foot with your arms.

4. Hold your hands either at your calf or ankle level, holding for 30 seconds before returning to the upright position then repeat for sets of repetitions before switching sides.

KEY POINTS TO REMEMBER:

• Relax slowly into positions.

• Concentrate on holding your abdominal muscles in during the duration of the exercise.

• Breathe deeply.

LOWER, MID AND UPPER BACK STRETCH

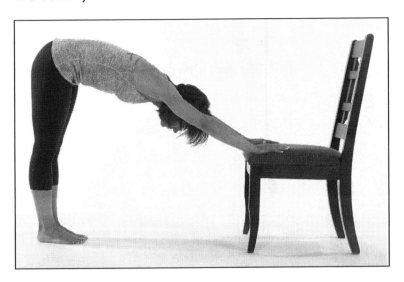

THE MOVEMENT:

1. Stand with your feet together with the chair in front of you about three feet away.

2. Next bend at your waist and place your hands on the chair keeping your arms straight and even with your ears.

3. Next lean forward with your upper body down toward your left foot with your arms.

4. Hold the position for 30 seconds before returning to the upright position then repeat for sets of repetitions before switching sides.

KEY POINTS TO REMEMBER:

• Relax slowly into positions.

• Allow the chair to aide you into the positions taking weight off your spine and joints.

• Concentrate on holding your abdominal muscles

LOWER, MID BACK AND LAT STRETCH

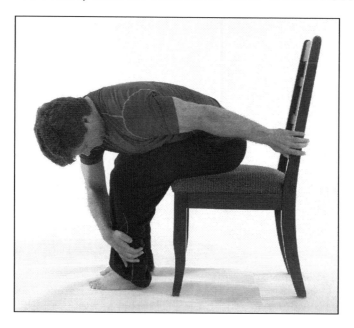

THE MOVEMENT:

1. Sitting upright on a chair with your feet together looking straight ahead.

2. Next lean forward with your upper body down while wrapping your right hand around your left ankle or calf.

3. Next place your left arm back and straight holding the back of the chair.

4. Hold this position for 30 seconds or longer before returning to the upright position then repeat for sets of repetitions before switching sides.

KEY POINTS TO REMEMBER:

• Don't twist your spine or over torque using upper body strength during the movement.

• Relax slowly into positions.

• Concentrate on holding your abdominal muscles in during the duration of the exercise.

• Breathe deeply.

SEATED HIP FLEXOR, GLUTES AND LOWER BACK STRETCH

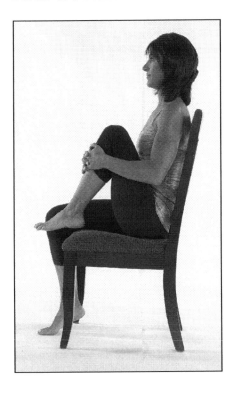

THE MOVEMENT:

1. Sitting upright on a chair with your feet shoulder width apart looking straight ahead.

2. Bending your left knee bring your left foot up and hugging your leg to your chest with both your hands.

3. Hold for 30 seconds or longer before returning your foot to the floor then repeat for sets of repetitions before switching sides.

KEY POINTS TO REMEMBER:

• Relax slowly into positions.

• Concentrate on holding your

LOWER, MID BACK, HIP AND GLUTE STRETCH

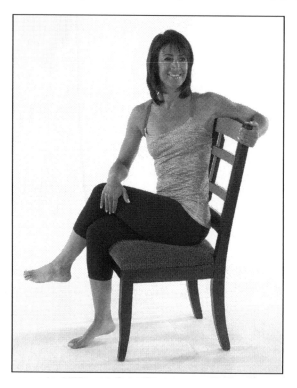

THE MOVEMENT:

1. Sitting upright on a chair with your feet shoulder width apart looking straight ahead.

2. Bending your left knee bring across your right leg while turning your upper body to the left placing your left hand on the back of the chair.

3. Next place your right hand across your left knee applying pressure to the outside of the left thigh area. Hold for 30 seconds or longer before returning your foot to the floor then repeat for sets of repetitions before switching sides.

KEY POINTS TO REMEMBER:

• Don't twist your spine or over torque using upper body strength during the movement.

• Relax slowly into positions.

• Concentrate on holding your abdominal muscles in during the duration of the exercise.

SHOULDER AND UPPER BACK STRETCH

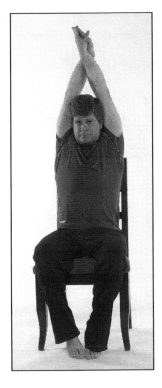

THE MOVEMENT:

1. Sitting upright on a chair with your feet together looking straight ahead.

2. Raise both your hands over head keeping your arms straight and inner lace your hands at the top of the movement. Maintain proper head position looking straight ahead at all times.

3. Next raise your shoulders up toward the ceiling as high as you can and hold for 30 seconds or longer before returning your arms down by your sides then repeat for sets of repetitions.

KEY POINTS TO REMEMBER:

• Concentrate on holding your abdominal muscles in during the duration of the exercise.

• Breathe deeply.

• Keep looking straight ahead.

UPPER BACK AND SHOULDER STRETCH

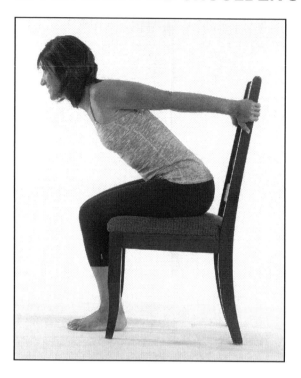

THE MOVEMENT:

1. Sitting upright on a chair with your feet together looking straight ahead.

2. Bring both your hands behind you keeping your arms straight and hold the back of the chair with your thumbs pointing down. Maintain proper head position looking straight ahead at all times.

3. Hold for 30 seconds or longer before returning your arms down by your sides then repeat for sets of repetitions.

KEY POINTS TO REMEMBER:

- Relax slowly into positions.

- Concentrate on holding your abdominal muscles in during the duration of the exercise.

UPPER AND MID BACK AND SHOULDER STRETCH

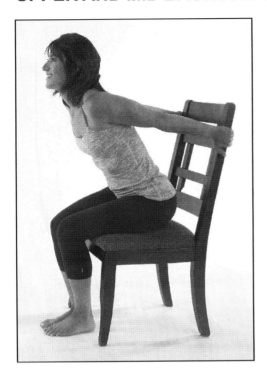

THE MOVEMENT:

1. Sitting upright on a chair with your feet together looking straight ahead.

2. Bring both your hands behind you keeping your arms straight and hold the back of the chair with your thumbs pointing down. Maintain proper head position looking straight ahead at all times.

3. Next raise your chest up as high as you comfortable can and hold for 30 seconds or longer before returning your arms down by your sides then repeat for sets of repetitions.

KEY POINTS TO REMEMBER:

• Relax slowly into positions.

• Concentrate on holding your abdominal muscles in during the duration of the exercise.

• Breathe deeply.

CHAPTER SUMMARY

- By using a chair or exercise ball you can enhance your flexibility safely and effectively without comprising your muscles or joints in the process.

- You are able to achieve greater range of motion without forcing your body into any uncomfortable positions or contortions to achieve your goals nor do you have to be born flexible.

- Maintain proper body alignment when moving through the exercises and preserve your muscle control while relaxing the other body parts that you are not stretching at that moment in time.

CHAPTER 7

DYNAMIC MOVING STRETCHES

ANKLE CIRCLES

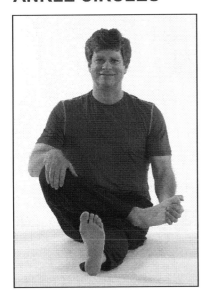

MUSCLE AND JOINT EMPHASIS:
Ankle joint and achillies tendon

THE POSITIONING:
Begin by sitting with your legs out stretched in front of you with your arms by your sides.

THE MOVEMENT:

1. Slowly raise your right foot and bending your knee allowing your foot to rest across your left thigh.

2. Grab your right foot with your left hand and place over your right ankle over the edge of your left thigh. Begin gently moving your foot in a counter clockwise circle with your left hand while relaxing your right ankle throughout the movement. Complete the movement after completing ten to fifteen rotations before reversing directions for the same amount of repetitions.

3. Immediately switch legs placing your left foot on your right thigh and repeat for the same amount of repetitions.

KEY POINTS TO REMEMBER:

- Focus on bringing your foot high enough up on your thigh to execute the movement.

- Concentrate on rotating your ankle joint during the duration of the exercise.

- Do not force your joint or muscle into the range of motion.

ANKLE AND HIP STRETCH

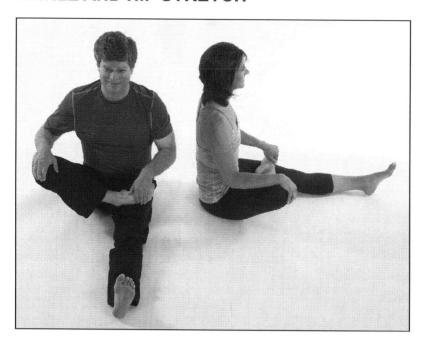

MUSCLE AND JOINT EMPHASIS:
Ankle joint, Achilles tendon, hip joint, and adductors.

THE POSITIONING:
Begin by sitting with your legs out stretched in front of you with your arms by your sides.

THE MOVEMENT:
1. Slowly raise your right foot and bending your knee allowing your foot to rest across your highest comfortable position on your left thigh.

2. Pull your right foot up so the bottom of your foot is turn up toward you with your left hand, while you use your right hand to press down onto your right bent thigh.

3. Slowly exhale as you relax into the stretch lowering your right knee down towards the floor and hold this position for three to five seconds before returning the knee to the beginning position. Rest for a few seconds maintain an upright posture breathing with your diaphragm in a nice relax pattern then repeat the exercise for additional five to ten repetitions.

4. Immediately switch legs placing your left foot on your right thigh and repeat for the same amount of repetitions.

ADVANCED MOVEMENT:

By incorporating resistance to the movement by stimulating more muscle fibers in step three above, you would use your right hand or forearm to apply resistance down onto your thigh while pulling up your right knee. By holding this isometric contraction for three seconds then relaxing your body will improve your range of motion. Do not over do the resistance part by doing too many repetitions after fatiguing out the muscle groups or your knee already touches the floor without resistance.

KEY POINTS TO REMEMBER:

- Focus on bringing your foot high enough up on your thigh to execute the movement while keeping an upright posture during the duration.

- Concentrate on turning your foot upward at the start of the exercise to ensure a complete stretch to the regions involved.

- Do not force your joint or muscle into the range of motion.

BUTTERFLIES

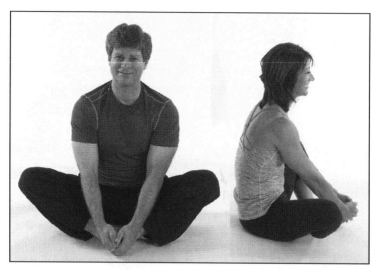

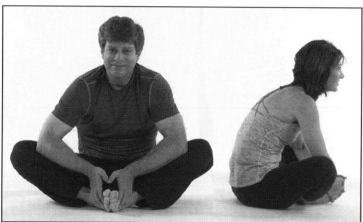

MUSCLE AND JOINT EMPHASIS:
Hips, knees, ankles inner and outer thighs

THE POSITIONING:
Begin by sitting with your legs bent at your knees with your feet together with your arms resting on your knees and hands on your feet.

THE MOVEMENT:
1. Slowly straighten your knees down toward the floor while holding your feet with your hands.

2. Slowly raise your knees up toward your shoulders then lower back down until your knees touch the floor. Complete ten to fifteen repetitions.

ADVANCED MOVEMENT:

Using resistance of your upper arms you can place your forearms or hands on your knees while pressing down onto them toward the floor while you squeeze your legs up against the resistance for three to five seconds then relax your legs down toward the floor then repeat.

KEY POINTS TO REMEMBER:

- Do not bounce your knees up and down in this position.

- Focus on bringing your feet as close to your body as possible before starting the movement.

- Concentrate on bring your knee down toward the floor during the duration of the exercise.

- Do not force your joint or muscle into the range of motion.

- When performing the advance move make sure you are applying equal amount of pressure on both sides of your body onto your legs.

TRIANGLE REACH STRETCH

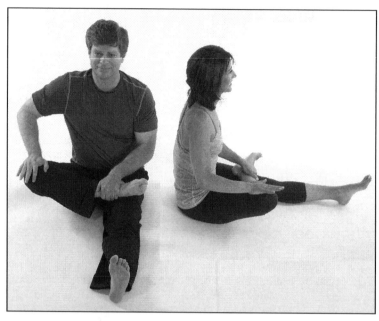

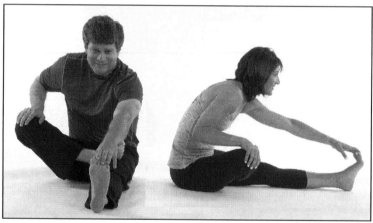

MUSCLE EMPHASIS:

Ankle joint, hamstrings hip joint, and adductors.

THE POSITIONING:

Begin with your right foot and bending your knee allowing your foot to rest across your highest comfortable position on your left thigh.

THE MOVEMENT:

1. Pull your right foot up so the bottom of your foot is turn up toward you while you use your right hand or forearm to press down onto your right bent thigh.

2. Reach with your left arm out toward your foot, if you can hold your toes or ankle to complete the movement. Hold for 10 to 20 seconds before switching legs placing your left foot on your right thigh and repeat for the same amount of repetitions.

ADVANCED MOVEMENT:

By incorporating resistance to the movement by stimulating more muscle fibers in step three above, you would use your right hand or forearm to apply resistance down onto your thigh while pulling up your right knee. By holding this isometric contraction for three seconds then relaxing your body will improve your range of motion. Do not over do the resistance part by doing too many repetitions after fatiguing out the muscle groups or your knee already touches the floor without resistance.

KEY POINTS TO REMEMBER:

- Focus on bringing your foot high enough up on your thigh to execute the movement while keeping an upright posture during the duration.

- Concentrate on turning your foot upward at the start of the exercise to ensure a complete stretch to the regions involved.

- Do not force your joint or muscle into the range of motion.

SEATED LEG HUG

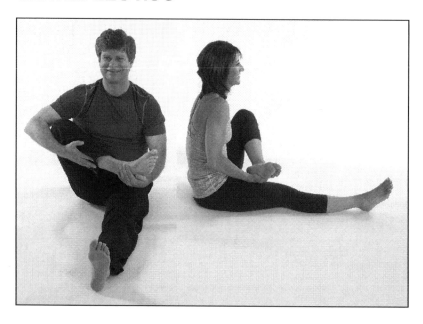

MUSCLE AND JOINT EMPHASIS:
Hips, knees, thighs and glutes.

THE POSITIONING:
Begin by sitting with your left leg out stretched in front of you and your right leg bent at the knee with your foot flat on the floor.

THE MOVEMENT:
1. Wrap both your hands around your bent right knee.

2. Slowly inhale as you draw your knee into your chest by pulling your hands towards your chest and hold this position exhaling for three to five seconds then relax and return your leg to the starting position and repeat a set of repetitions before switching legs.

KEY POINTS TO REMEMBER:
- Do not pull your knee up and off the floor during the movement. Rather glide your foot across toward you.

- Focus on maintaining a relaxed upright posture throughout the movement.

- Don't round yourself forward over your knee during the exercise.

SQUAT ONE

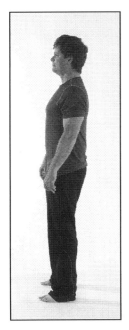 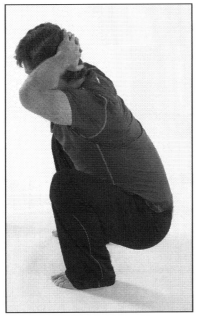

MUSCLE AND JOINT EMPHASIS:
Hips, knees, thighs, glutes, upper back and shoulder muscles.

THE POSITIONING:
Begin by standing with your feet shoulder width apart and your hands behind your head with your elbows bent.

THE MOVEMENT:
1. Slowly lower yourself down bending your knees as far as you can go while maintaining your heels on the floor throughout the movement.

2. Slowly bend your head forward towards the floor in the end position feeling the stretch in the upper back area and hold this position for three to five seconds before returning to the upright standing position. Then repeat the movement again for a set of repetitions.

KEY POINTS TO REMEMBER:
- Maintain an upright posture while squatting down until you are at your farthest depth.

- Focus on keeping your heels on the ground.

PLIE SQUATS

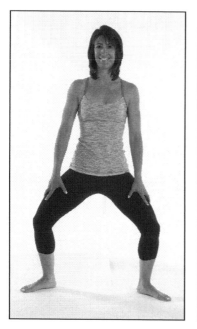 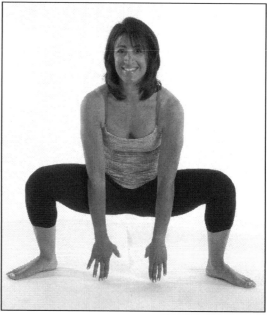

MUSCLE AND JOINT EMPHASIS:
Hips, knees, thighs, glutes, upper back and shoulder muscles.

THE POSITIONING:
Begin by standing with your feet greater than shoulder width apart and pleated outward with your arms down by your side.

THE MOVEMENT:

1. Slowly lower yourself down bending your knees as far as you can go while maintaining your heels on the floor throughout the movement.

2. Maintain your balance by placing your hands in front of you and try to touch the floor with your hands at the end position. Then repeat the movement again for a set of repetitions.

KEY POINTS TO REMEMBER:

- Maintain an upright posture while squatting down until you are at your farthest depth.

- Focus on keeping your heels on the ground.

STANDING BENT OVER ARM HOLD

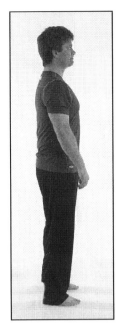 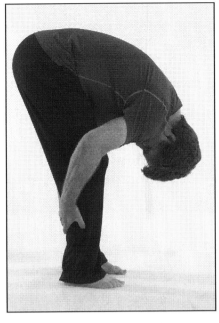

MUSCLE AND JOINT EMPHASIS:
Hips, Hamstrings, glutes, upper, mid back, and shoulder muscles.

THE POSITIONING:
Begin by standing with your feet shoulder width a part with your arms relaxed by your sides.

THE MOVEMENT:
1. Slowly Lean forward at the waist as you bend your knees slightly as you allow your arms to hanging down toward the floor.

2. Next slowly place your hands behind your ankles or calves and hold yourself in this position for three to five seconds before returning to the upright position and repeat a set of repetitions.

KEY POINTS TO REMEMBER:
- Relax your upper arms and shoulders during the movement; do not pull yourself down toward the ground at any time.

- Relax and breathe deeply during the stretch.

SEATED ARM TURTLE STRETCH

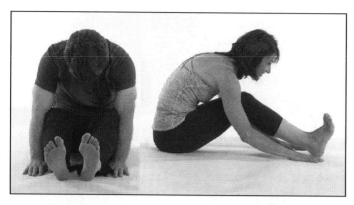

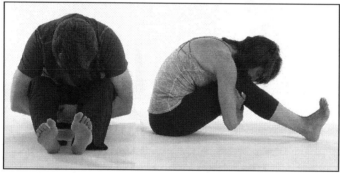

MUSCLE AND JOINT EMPHASIS:
Hips, Hamstrings, glutes, upper, mid, lower back, and shoulder muscles.

THE POSITIONING:
Begin by sitting with your feet shoulder width a part and your legs outstretched in front of you with your arms relaxed by your sides.

THE MOVEMENT:
1. Slowly Lean forward at the waist as you bend your knees as you allow your arms to go under your knees while your hands touch the floor.

2. Resting your upper body on top of your legs this position for 10 to 30 seconds before returning to the upright position and repeat a set of repetitions.

KEY POINTS TO REMEMBER:
- Relax your upper arms and shoulders during the movement, do not pull yourself down.

- Hold your stomach muscles in throughout the exercise.

ADVANCED BALANCE SQUAT PIRIFORMIS STRETCH

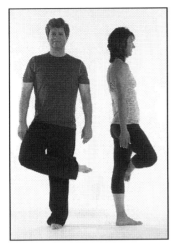 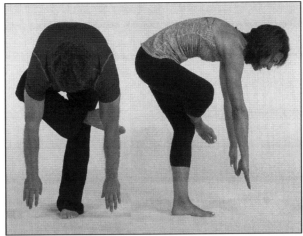

MUSCLE AND JOINT EMPHASIS:
Piriformis, hips, hamstrings, glutes, and lower back muscles.

THE POSITIONING:
Begin by standing with your feet shoulder width a part with a slight bend in your knees with your arms relaxed by your sides.

THE MOVEMENT:
1. Slowly place your right leg with your knee bent resting on top of your left thigh just above the knee. Lean forward at your waist as you bend your left leg as you allow your arms to go down to as your hands touch the floor.

2. Next hold yourself in this position for three to five seconds before returning to the upright position and repeat a set of repetitions.

KEY POINTS TO REMEMBER:
- Maintain an upright posture with your shoulders back at the start of the exercise.

- Maintain your balance by moving your feet shoulder width apart at the start of the movement.

- If you are unable to touch the floor with your hands you can do the movement with a support of a chair in front of you by resting your hands on the chair until your flexibility improves.

BACKWARDS BEND

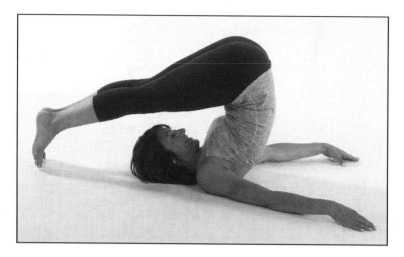

MUSCLE AND JOINT EMPHASIS:
Hips, hamstrings, glutes, and lower back muscles.

THE POSITIONING:
Begin by sitting with your feet shoulder width a part and your legs outstretched in front of you with your arms relaxed by your sides.

THE MOVEMENT:
1. Slowly raise your legs up keep your feet together as you bend your knees toward your chest then roll backwards keeping your arms down by your side.

2. Next bring your feet toward your head while straightening your legs down and try to touch the floor with your feet.

3. After holding the position for three to five seconds slowly return to the starting position and repeat for a set.

KEY POINTS TO REMEMBER:
- Do not do this movement if you have neck or back issues
- Relax your lower back during the movement.
- Pull your stomach muscles in throughout the exercise.
- Maintain a steady rhythm in your speed during the exercise.
- You can place a chair behind you and place your feet on it.

LYING LEG AND PIRIFORMIS STRETCH

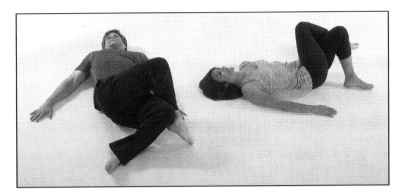

MUSCLE AND JOINT EMPHASIS:
Hips, piriformis, hamstrings, glutes, and lower back muscles.

THE POSITIONING:
Begin by lying on the floor with your knees bent and feet flat on the floor and your arms down by your side.

THE MOVEMENT:
1. Slowly raise your right foot up and place it onto your left knee with your right knee bent out to the side.

2. Then bring your right foot down toward your left side of your hip and hold your leg with your leg in this position.

3. Next take your right hand and press down onto your right knee feeling the stretch along your leg and hip regions hold this position for three to five seconds slowly return to the starting position and repeat for a set before switching to the opposite leg.

KEY POINTS TO REMEMBER:
- Relax your Hips and lower back during the movement.

- Maintain a steady rhythm in your speed during the exercise.

- Pull with your foot into position as far and as comfortable as you can.

LYING LEG AND PIRIFORMIS STRETCH #2

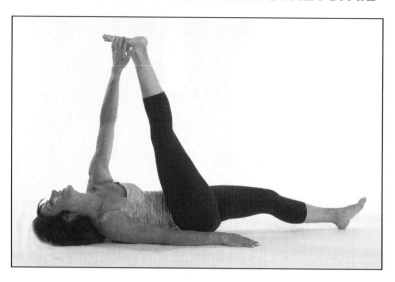

MUSCLE AND JOINT EMPHASIS:
Hips, piriformis, hamstrings, glutes, and lower back muscles.

THE POSITIONING:
Begin by lying on the floor with your back flat on the floor and your arms down by your side.

THE MOVEMENT:

1. Slowly raise your right foot up with knee bent and hold onto your foot with your left hand. Keeping your left knee bent and foot flat on the floor.

2. Next bring your right leg up and toward your chest as you use your left arm to guide your leg up then straighten at the top of the movement. Hold this position for three to five seconds then slowly return to the starting position and repeat for a set before switching to the opposite leg.

3. Advance movement straighten your left leg once you reach the top position with your right leg for a greater stretch in both legs.

KEY POINTS TO REMEMBER:

- Hold your stomach muscles in throughout the exercise.

- Maintain a steady rhythm in your speed during the exercise.

- Bring your leg into position as far and as comfortable as you can.

- Hold onto the outside of your foot.

The next movements build upon each other and are highly recommended that you follow them in this sequence to achieve optimum flexibility.

LYING HALF BUTTERFLY WITH RESISTANCE

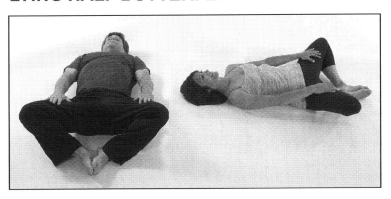

MUSCLE AND JOINT EMPHASIS:
Hips, adductors, abductors, hamstrings, piriformis, glutes, and lower back muscles.

THE POSITIONING:
Begin by lying down with your lower back flat and your knees bent and the bottom of your feet together and your hands resting on the floor.

THE MOVEMENT:
1. Drop your legs down toward the floor while you pulling in your abdominal muscles.

2. Then take your hands and press down against your thighs for an isometric contraction of three to five seconds before relaxing and lowering your legs down further without resistance. Slowly relax and repeat for a complete set.

KEY POINTS TO REMEMBER:
- Keep your back flat.
- Relax your Hips and lower back during the movement.
- Hold your stomach muscles in throughout the exercise.

SEATED SINGLE LEG STRETCH

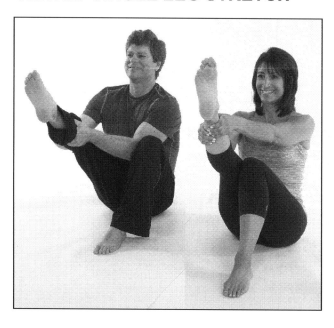

MUSCLE AND JOINT EMPHASIS:
Hips, Hamstrings, pirformis, glutes, and lower back muscles.

THE POSITIONING:
Begin by sitting on the floor with your legs out stretched and your resting at your right knee or below.

THE MOVEMENT:
1. Bend your left knee and rest your left foot flat on the floor.

2. Keeping your right leg straight, raise your leg up while holding onto your right ankle or calf with your hands.

3. Now straighten your back more and pull your right leg towards your chest while pulling in your abdominals.

4. Hold for two to three seconds in this top position before lowering your right leg back to the floor and repeat for a set before switching to the opposite leg.

KEY POINTS TO REMEMBER:
• Keep your back straight during the movement as much as possible.

• Maintain a steady rhythm in your speed during the exercise.

• Keep your head up and looking straight during the exercise.

SEATED LEG SPLITS

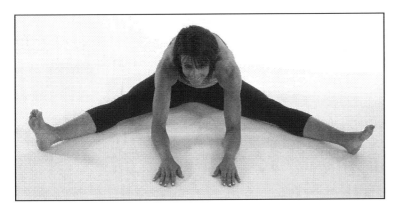

MUSCLE AND JOINT EMPHASIS:
Hips, hamstrings, piriformis, glutes, and lower back muscles.

THE POSITIONING:
Begin by sitting on the floor with your legs out stretched to the side and your arms by your sides.

THE MOVEMENT:

1. Place your hands behind your back without stretched arms and slowly move your legs farther apart as you push with your hands.

2. Then place your forearms on the floor in front of you as you lean forward with a straight back. Holding this position for three to five seconds before returning to the upright position with your arms by your side then repeat.

KEY POINTS TO REMEMBER:

- Do not round your back when performing this movement.

- Pull in and contract your abdominal muscles throughout the exercise.

SEATED LEG SPLITS WITH UPPER BODY CIRCLES

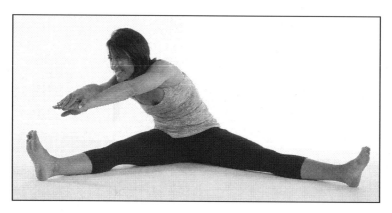

MUSCLE AND JOINT EMPHASIS:
Hips, hamstrings, piriformis, glutes, and lower back muscles.

THE POSITIONING:
Begin by sitting on the floor with your legs out stretched to the side and your arms by your sides.

THE MOVEMENT:
1. Place your hands behind your back without stretched arms and slowly move your legs farther apart as you push with your hands.

2. Next place your arms out stretched and over your head inter locking your fingers keeping your arms straight. Then start clockwise bending at your waist keeping the back straight throughout the movement and lean towards your right foot with your hands and sweep across toward your left foot and back up to the top and repeat for a set before switching to opposite direction and repeat for a set.

KEY POINTS TO REMEMBER:
- Pull in and contract your abdominal muscles throughout the exercise
- Reach out as far as you can with your arms throughout the exercise

SIDE LUNGE STRETCH

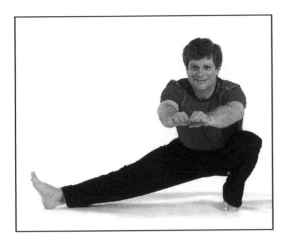

MUSCLE AND JOINT EMPHASIS:
Adductors, abductors, hips, hamstrings, glutes, piriformis, lower and mid back muscles, and shoulder region.

THE POSITIONING:
Begin by standing with your feet shoulder width a part with a slight bend in your knees with your arms relaxed by your sides.

THE MOVEMENT:
1. Slowly shift your weight onto your left leg while bending your left knee as you turn your right foot up and keep your right leg straight. Lean forward slightly at your waist and bring your arms forward without touching your hands on the floor. Hold for three to five seconds before returning to the upright position and repeat on the opposite side.

KEY POINTS TO REMEMBER:
- Maintain an upright posture with your shoulders back at the start of the exercise

- Maintain your balance by moving your arms forward

- If you are unable to keep your balance, place your hands on the floor lightly during the exercise until you are able to perform the movement without supporting yourself with your arms.

SEATED HIP STRETCH

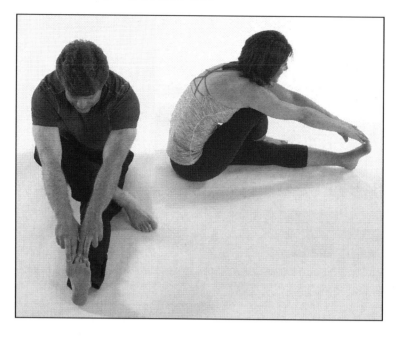

MUSCLE AND JOINT EMPHASIS:
Hip joint, abductors, TFL band and lower back muscles

THE POSITIONING:
Begin by sitting with your legs out stretched in front of you with your arms by your sides.

THE MOVEMENT:
1. Next bring your right foot over your left leg above your knee height. Maintain an upright position throughout the movement keeping the back straight.

1. Next place your hands in front of you and slowly lean forward until you touch and hold your toes or ankle and hold for three to five seconds before returning to an upright position then repeat. Immediately switch legs after completing a set.

KEY POINTS TO REMEMBER:
- Focus on relaxing into the stretch rather than pulling yourself into any one position.

- Do not force your joint or muscle into the range of motion.

SEATED LEG CROSS STRETCH

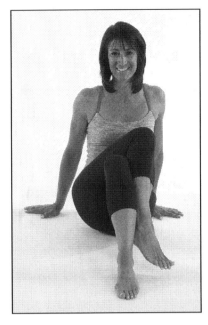 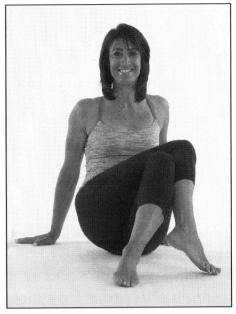

MUSCLE AND JOINT EMPHASIS:
Hip joint, abductors, TFL band, hamstrings and lower back muscles

THE POSITIONING:
Begin by crossing your right leg over your left leg at the left knee and place your right foot around your left calf or ankle with your arms by your sides

THE MOVEMENT:
1. Next drop your right leg over toward your left side trying to touch the floor with your right knee while maintaining an upright position throughout the exercise. Hold for three to five seconds before turning your right leg to the right and down and then hold this position for three to five seconds before returning to the center then repeat. Switch legs after completing a set.

KEY POINTS TO REMEMBER:
- Do not force your joint or muscle into the range of motion.
- Maintain an upright posture.

SEATED PIRIFORMIS STRETCH

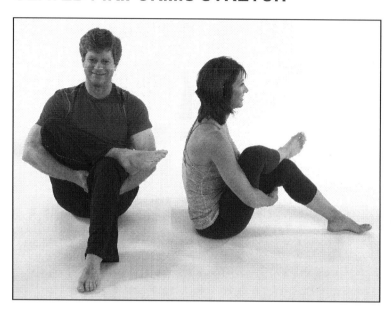

MUSCLE AND JOINT EMPHASIS:
Piriformis, hip joint, abductors, adductors, TFL band, hamstrings and lower back muscles

THE POSITIONING:
Begin by sitting with your knees bent and your feet flat on the floor with your arms by your sides.

THE MOVEMENT:
1. Begin by sitting with your knees bent and your feet flat on the floor with your arms by your sides.

2. Place your arms around your right and left leg interlacing your hands under your left knee with an upright posture. Pull your right leg up toward your chest and hold for three to five seconds before turning your right leg the floor and repeat for a set before switching to the opposite leg.

KEY POINTS TO REMEMBER:
- Concentrate on pulling in you abdominal muscles during the duration of the exercise.

- Adjust foot position to vary the stretch by increasing the stretch by bring your foot closer to your body on the floor or farther away if you have less flexibility.

LYING CHEST OPENER STRETCH

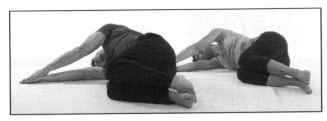

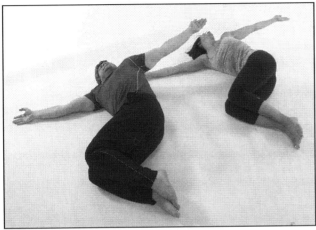

MUSCLE AND JOINT EMPHASIS:
Chest, anterior deltoid, upper and lower back muscles

THE POSITIONING:
Begin by lying with your legs out stretched in front of you with your arms by
your sides.

THE MOVEMENT:
1. Bend your knees while turning on your right side and bring them up toward
   your waistline forming a ninety degree with your torso.

2. Next open upwards by bring your left arm across your body behind your
   back and place your hand on the floor at or above your head height if you
   can. Turn your head toward the ceiling or left arm as you move through the
   motion allowing you to stretch your neck muscles as well. Hold for three
   to five seconds before returning to the start then repeat for a set before
   switching sides.

KEY POINTS TO REMEMBER:
- Do not twist yourself into any position rather focus on the
  muscles stretching.

PIRIFORMIS STRETCH

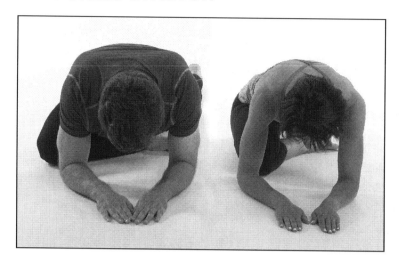

MUSCLE AND JOINT EMPHASIS:
Hip joint, piriformis, abductors, adductors, TFL band, hamstrings and lower back muscles

THE POSITIONING:
Begin by kneeling on the floor with your hands on the floor supporting your upper body weight.

THE MOVEMENT:

1. Go into the push up position and next bring your right leg forward with your knee bent with your right foot to your left side even near your left elbow.

2. Next relax your upper body over your right leg, resting on your forearm on the floor and keep your left foot instep flat on the floor throughout the movement return to the upright position then repeat before switching to the opposite leg for a set.

KEY POINTS TO REMEMBER:

- Concentrate on pulling in you abdominal muscles during the duration of the exercise.

- Do not force your joint or muscle into the range of motion.

PIRIFORMIS STRETCH WITH QUAD STRETCH

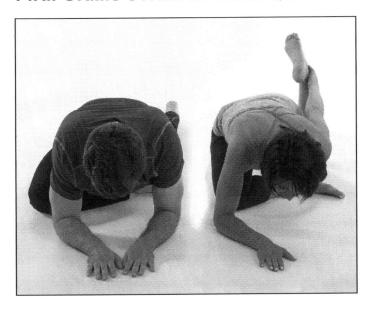

MUSCLE AND JOINT EMPHASIS:
Hip joint, hip flexors, pirfomis, abductors, adductors, TFL band, hamstrings and quadriceps muscles

THE POSITIONING:
Begin by kneeling on the floor with your hands on the floor supporting your upper body weight.

THE MOVEMENT:

1. Go into the push up position and next bring your right leg forward with your knee bent with your right foot to your left side even near your left elbow.

2. Next relax your upper body over your right leg, resting on your forearm on the floor and keep your left foot in step flat on the floor throughout the movement. Next bend your left knee and bring your left foot toward your lower back.

3. Next hold your left foot with your left hand and hold this position for three to five seconds before returning to the upright position then repeat before switching to the opposite leg for a set.

KEY POINTS TO REMEMBER:

- Don't arch your back when reaching behind to hold your foot during the exercise.

PIRIFORMIS STRETCH WITH SIDE KICK STRETCH

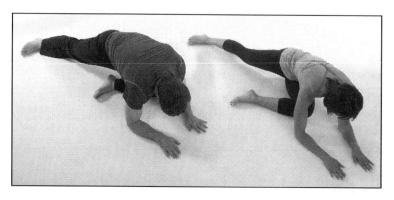

MUSCLE AND JOINT EMPHASIS:
Hip joint, hip flexors, glutes, piriformis, abductors, adductors, TFL band, hamstrings and lower back muscles

THE POSITIONING:
Begin by kneeling on the floor with your hands on the floor supporting your upper body weight.

THE MOVEMENT:
1. Go into the push up position and next bring your left leg forward with your knee bent with your right foot to your right side even near your right elbow.

2. Next relax your upper body over your left leg, resting on your forearms on the floor.

3. Next turn your left foot sideways with your foot edge flat on the floor throughout the movement and hold for three to five seconds.

4. Return to the upright position then repeat before switching to the opposite leg for a set.

KEY POINTS TO REMEMBER:
• Don't twist your back when reaching across with your arm, instead feel the stretch acquiring at your upper body.

KNEELING QUAD AND SIDE TURN STRETCH

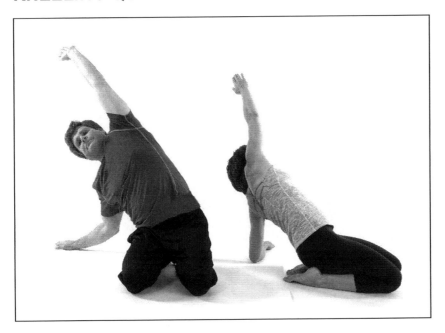

MUSCLE AND JOINT EMPHASIS:
Quadriceps, hip flexors, obliques, lats, lower back, and, shoulders muscles

THE POSITIONING:
Begin by kneeling with your knees bent and your feet underneath you with your arms by your sides.

THE MOVEMENT:
1. Lean back at your waist while maintaining an upright posture. Pull in your abdominal muscles while doing so. Place your arm slightly behind and off to the side resting on your elbow for support and gently raise your opposite arm up and over your head toward your side, reaching as far back as you can until you feel a stretch in your front thighs and shoulder muscles.

2. Hold for three to five seconds before returning to the upright position then repeat on the opposite side.

KEY POINTS TO REMEMBER:
- Do not perform if you have any knee issues.
- Adjust your arm placement on the floor to further increase the stretch.

SEATED HURDLER STRETCH WITH A PUSH

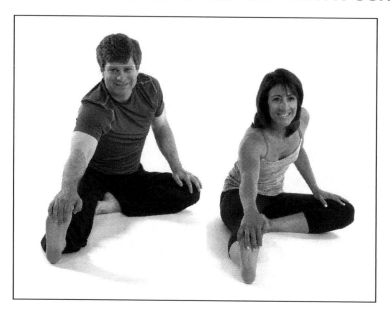

MUSCLE AND JOINT EMPHASIS:
Hip joint, hamstrings, obliques, and back and shoulder muscles

THE POSITIONING:
Begin by sitting with your right leg out stretched to front of you. Next bend your left knee and bring your left foot against your right upper thigh with your arms by your sides.

THE MOVEMENT:
1. Flex your toes back toward yourself while bending forward toward your right leg at your waist as you pull in your stomach muscles and reach with your right arm out over your right foot before resting your hand either on your foot or ankle. Next place your left hand on your left thigh above your knee and press down.

2. Hold for three to five seconds pushing against your thigh. Then relax further into the stretch before returning to the upright position then repeat a set before switching sides.

KEY POINTS TO REMEMBER:
- Involve your whole body in the stretch.

- Do not force your joint or muscle into the range of motion.

OLD SCHOOL HURDLER STRETCH

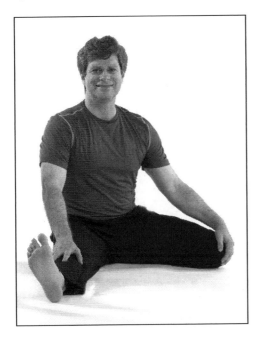

MUSCLE AND JOINT EMPHASIS:
Hip joint, hamstrings, obliques, and back and shoulder muscles

THE POSITIONING:
Begin by sitting with your right leg out stretched to front of you. Next bend your left knee and bring your left foot behind you adjusting the distance to your comfort level of the stretch.

THE MOVEMENT:
1. Flex your toes back toward yourself while bending forward toward your right leg at your waist as you pull in your stomach muscles and reach with your right arm out over your right foot before resting your hand either on your foot or ankle. Next place your left hand on your knee.

2. Hold for three to five seconds before returning to the upright position then repeat a set before switching sides.

KEY POINTS TO REMEMBER:
- Only do if you have no knee pain or issues.

- Do not force your joint or muscle into the range of motion.

SEATED HURDLER STRETCH WITH A LEAN

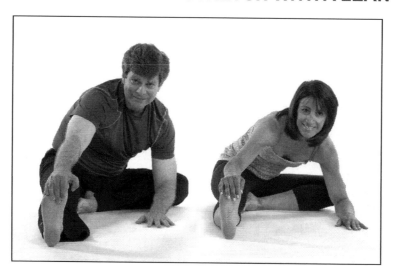

MUSCLE AND JOINT EMPHASIS:
Hip joint, hamstrings, obliques, and back and shoulder muscles

THE POSITIONING:
Begin by sitting with your right leg out stretched to front of you. Next bend your left knee and bring your left foot against your right upper thigh with your arms by your sides.

THE MOVEMENT:
1. Flex your toes back toward yourself while bending forward toward your right leg at your waist as you pull in your stomach muscles and reach with your right arm out over your right foot before resting your hand either on your foot or ankle. Next place your left hand or forearm on the floor.

2. Next move your left arm forward staying low in the movement until you cannot go any further.

3. Hold for three to five seconds pushing against your thigh. Then relax further into the stretch before returning to the upright position then repeat a set before switching sides.

KEY POINTS TO REMEMBER:
- Involve your whole body in the stretch.
- Do not force your joint or muscle into the range of motion.

ADDUCTOR AND SHOULDER STRETCH

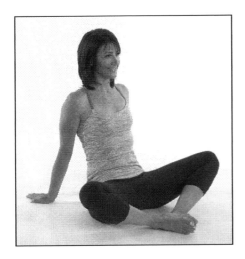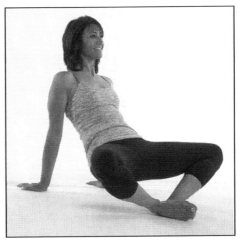

MUSCLE AND JOINT EMPHASIS:
Hip joint, adductors, back and shoulder muscles

THE POSITIONING:
Begin by sitting with your legs bent at your knees with your feet together with your arms shoulder width apart resting behind you with your fingers pointing away from you. Next lower your knees toward the floor as far as you can hold this position.

THE MOVEMENT:
1. Next lift yours elf off the floor while pressing your legs down, keep your legs in place, hold for three to five seconds before returning to the upright position then repeat for a set of repetitions.

KEY POINTS TO REMEMBER:
- Do not raise yourself up if you have any shoulder issues.
- Involve your whole body in the stretch.
- Do not force your joint or muscle into the range of motion.

SHOULDER REACH STRETCH

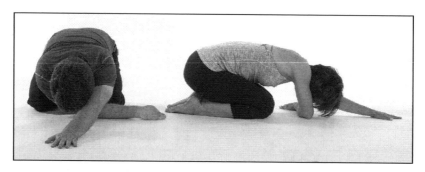

MUSCLE AND JOINT EMPHASIS:
Quadriceps, back and shoulder muscles

THE POSITIONING:
Begin by kneeling sitting on your heels if you can with your feet together with your arms shoulder width outstretched in front of you with your hands on the floor as far as you can and hold this position three to five seconds.

THE MOVEMENT:
1. Next bend your right arm and slide it under your left shoulder and reach as far as you can and, hold for three to five seconds before returning to both arms stretched out in front position then repeat for a set of repetitions.

KEY POINTS TO REMEMBER:
- Do not perform kneeling if you have any knee or leg issues.
- Involve your whole body in the stretch.
- Do not force your joint or muscle into the range of motion.

CHAPTER SUMMARY

- In this chapter you have learned to break through your flexibility barriers with this very effective stretching routine that will increase your overall flexibility and conditioning while toning your muscles using your own body resistance.

- Having gained flexibility from the other stretches in the earlier chapters, you built a more advanced form of stretching.

- Using force to enhance your overall flexibility takes you into another dimension of exercising. With practice you will learn to truly link the mind-body connection by improving your senses using these movements and overcome your limitations in a step-by-step method. Remember to maintain a steady rhythm in your speed during the exercise.

CHAPTER 8

SEQUENCE STRETCHES
WHEN YOU NEED TO BYPASS A STICKING POINT IN YOUR FLEXIBILITY

STANDING QUAD-HAM STRETCH

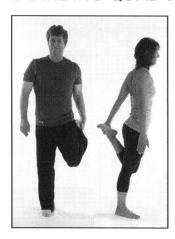
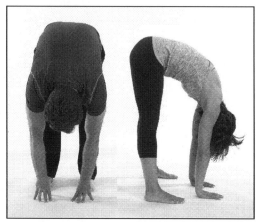

MUSCLE AND JOINT EMPHASIS:
Hips, hamstrings, glutes, upper, mid back, and shoulder muscles

THE POSITIONING:
Begin by standing with your feet shoulder width a part with your arms relaxed by your sides.

THE MOVEMENT:
1. Bend your left knee and hold your left foot with your left hand while bringing your foot toward your lower back feeling the stretch in your front thigh. Hold for three to five seconds before returning your left foot to the floor.

2. Next slowly Lean forward at the waist as keeping your knees straight as possible as you press your hands down toward the floor. Hold for three to five seconds before returning to the upright position and repeat with the right leg to complete sequence.

KEY POINTS TO REMEMBER:
• Relax into the movements; do not pull hard on your knee joint at any time.

• You can bend your knees slightly when bending over to start and as you warm up you can straighten your knees during the stretch.

KNEELING FRONT STRETCH

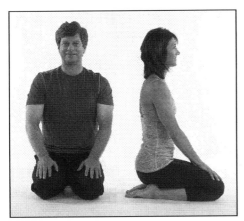 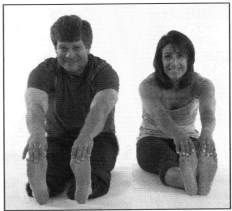

MUSCLE AND JOINT EMPHASIS:
Hips, quads, hamstrings, glutes, and lower back muscles

THE POSITIONING:
Begin by kneeling with your knees bent and your feet underneath you with your hands resting on your thighs.

THE MOVEMENT:
1. Seat back further onto your heels while maintaining an upright posture. Pull in your abdominal muscles while doing so. Hold for three to five seconds.

2. Next bring your legs out in front of you with your knees straight. Then reach with your hands and either hold your ankles or feet.

3. Lean forward further as you flex your toes back toward you and hold for three to five seconds before returning to the kneeling position then repeat.

KEY POINTS TO REMEMBER:
- Keep your back straight during the movement as much as possible.
- Maintain a steady rhythm in your speed during the exercise.
- Keep your head up and looking straight during the exercise.

QAUD-LYING HAMSTRING LEG STRETCH

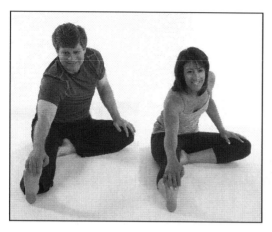 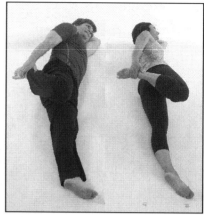

MUSCLE AND JOINT EMPHASIS:
Hips, hamstrings, glutes, and lower back muscles

THE POSITIONING:
Begin by sitting on the floor with your legs out stretched your arms by your side.

THE MOVEMENT:
1. Bend your left knee and rest your left foot against your right inner thigh on the floor.

2. Keeping your right leg straight, reach out and forward with your right hand holding onto your right foot or calf with your hand. Next place your left hand on your left knee and press your knee down further toward the floor.

3. Now straighten your back more lifting up your chest while maintaining your hand positions and pull in your abdominals.

4. Hold for two to three seconds in this position before turning onto your side into the lying quad stretch position with the same leg then repeat switching to the opposite leg for the same number of repetitions and sets.

KEY POINTS TO REMEMBER:
- Keep your back straight during the movement as much as possible.
- Maintain a steady rhythm in your speed during the exercise.
- Keep your head up and looking straight during the exercise.

HURDLER-SIDE ELBOW REACH LEG STRETCH

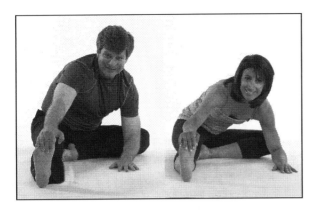

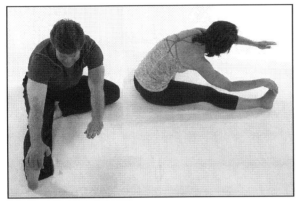

MUSCLE AND JOINT EMPHASIS:
Hip joint, hamstrings, obliques, and back and shoulder muscles

THE POSITIONING:
Begin by sitting with your right leg out stretched to front of you. Next bend your left knee and bring your left foot against your right upper thigh with your arms by your sides.

THE MOVEMENT:
1. Flex your toes back toward yourself while bending forward toward your right leg at your waist as you pull in your stomach muscles and reach with your right arm out over your right foot before resting your hand either on your foot or ankle. Next place your left hand or forearm on the floor.

2. Next move your left arm up and forward reaching out until you cannot go any further. Then return to the upright position then repeat on opposite side switching between sides throughout the set.

SEATED LEG TUCK STRETCH

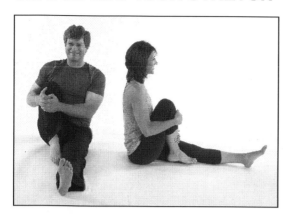

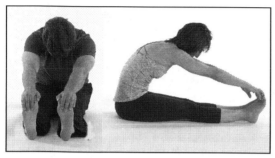

MUSCLE AND JOINT EMPHASIS:
Hip flexors, Hamstrings, glutes, and lower back muscles

THE POSITIONING:
Begin by sitting on the floor with your legs out stretched.

THE MOVEMENT:
1. Bend your right knee and rest your right foot flat on the floor.

2. Pulling your knee up into your chest and hold for three to five seconds.

3. Next lower and straighten your right leg then reach forward with your arms holding onto your ankles or feet while looking down. Hold three to five seconds before switching to your left leg pulling into your chest alternating for the remaining set of repetitions.

KEY POINTS TO REMEMBER:
• Maintain a steady rhythm in your speed during the exercise.

• You can bend your knees slightly at the beginning as you warm up to increase your range of motion.

KNEELING SIDE-SHOULDER REACH STRETCH

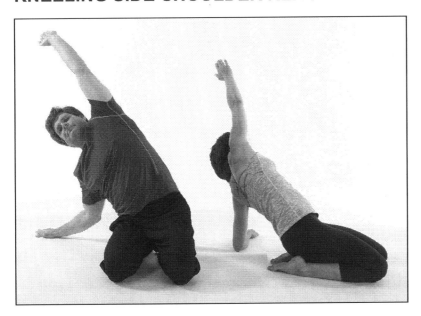

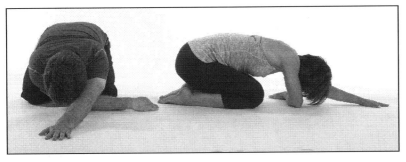

MUSCLE AND JOINT EMPHASIS:
Quadriceps, hip-flexors, obliques, back and shoulder muscles

THE POSITIONING:
Begin by kneeling with your knees bent and your feet underneath you with your arms by your sides.

THE MOVEMENT:

1. Lean back at your waist while maintaining an upright posture. Pull in your abdominal muscles while doing so. Place your right arm slightly behind and off to the side resting on your elbow for support and gently raise your opposite arm up and over your head toward your side, reaching as far back as you can until you feel a stretch in your front thighs and shoulder muscles.

2. Hold for three to five seconds

3. Next Lean forward bending at your waist as you slide your right arm under your left shoulder and reach as far as you can with your right and left hands. Hold for three to five seconds before returning to upright position then repeat the whole movement on the opposite side Alternating repetitions throughout the set.

CHAPTER 9

SUGGESTED STRETCHING ROUTINES FOR SPORTS

Now that you have learned the stretches and the proper breathing, it's time to put together a routine. This chapter will give you a number of options at each level, for the beginner to the more advanced athlete, giving guidance and direction for a complete full body stretching program. Included in this chapter are routines for those short on time that need a full body routine, as well as those who need to focus on a particular region for a given sport.

I have clustered these activities together based on my clinical experience with athletes in these chosen sports. Feel free to interchange the options. Remember it's all about variety.

BASEBALL, TENNIS, GOLF, BOWLING, CRICKET STRETCHING ROUTINES

These movements are geared towards balancing out your body, especially for any sport involving one side of your body more than the other.

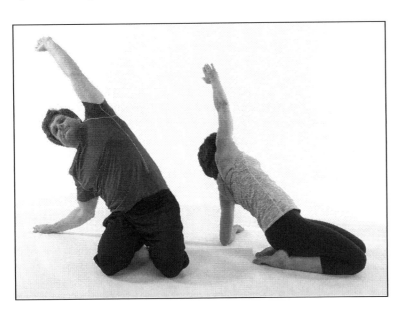

BASEBALL, TENNIS, GOLF, BOWLING, CRICKET STRETCHING ROUTINES CONTINUED

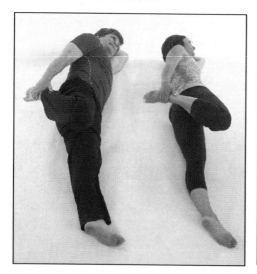 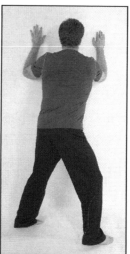

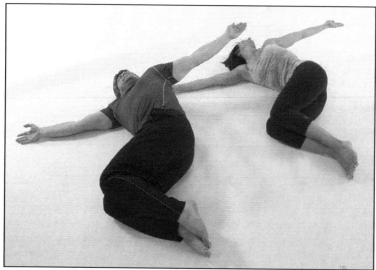

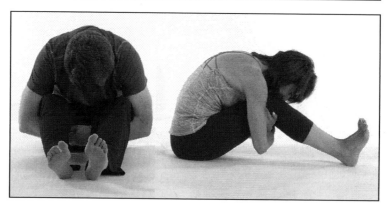

**BASEBALL, TENNIS, GOLF, BOWLING, CRICKET STRETCHING
ROUTINES CONTINUED**

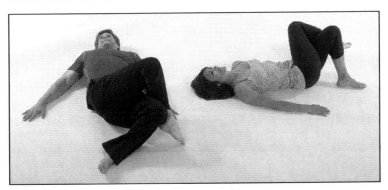

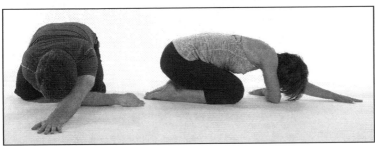

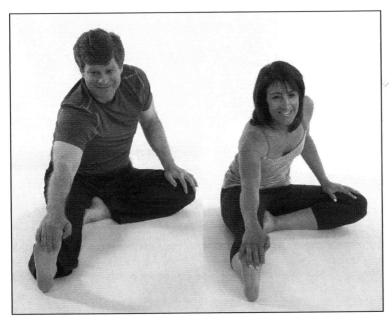

FOOTBALL, LA CROSS, ROWING, SWIMMING STRETCHING ROUTINES

These movements are geared towards any sport that uses rhythmic patterns.

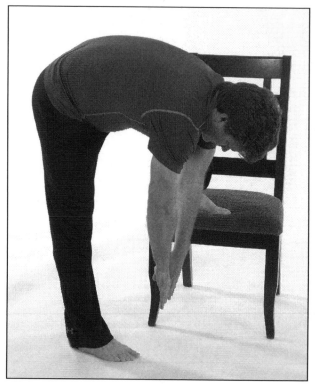
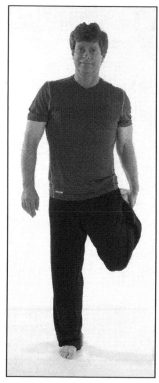
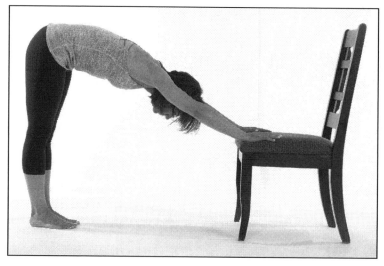

FOOTBALL, LA CROSS, ROWING, SWIMMING STRETCHING ROUTINES CONTINUED

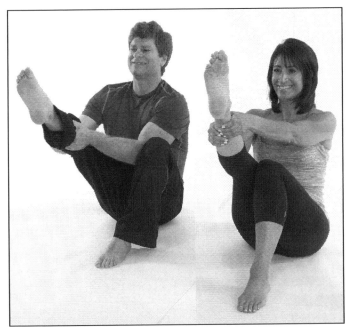 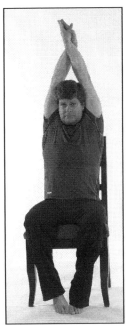

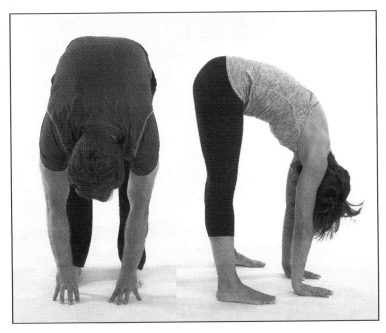

**FOOTBALL, LA CROSS, ROWING, SWIMMING STRETCHING
ROUTINES CONTINUED**

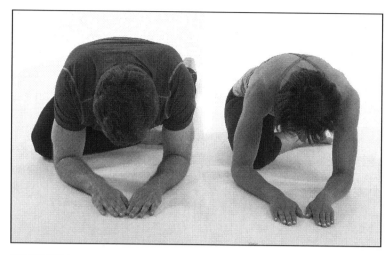

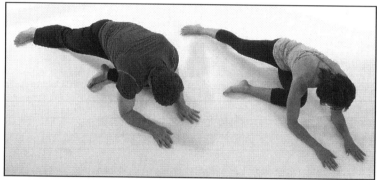

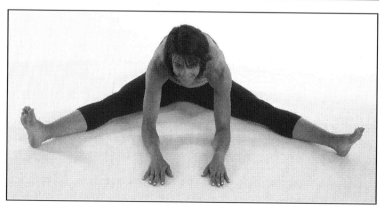

BODYBUILDING, CROSS TRAINING, POWER-LIFTING STRETCHING ROUTINES

These movements can be incorporated between resting sets.

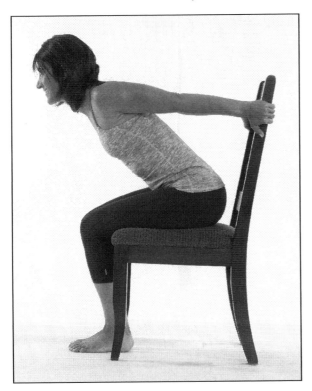

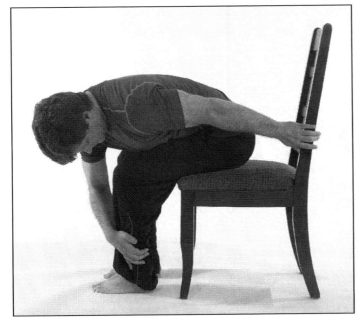

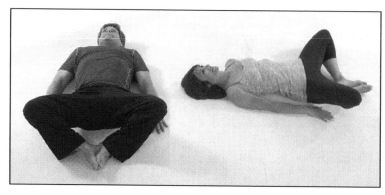

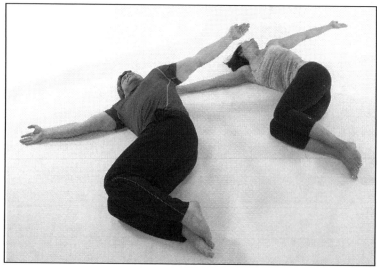

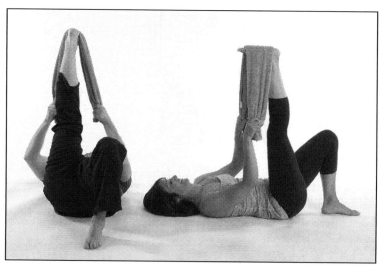

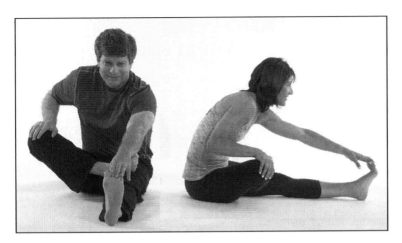

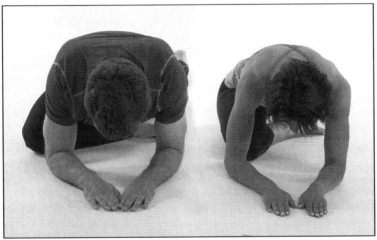

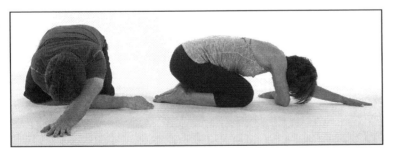

BODYBUILDING, CROSS TRAINING, POWER-LIFTING STRETCHING ROUTINES CONTINUED

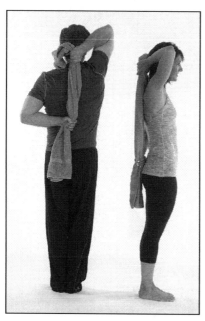

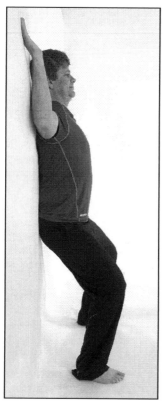

CYCLING, SOCCER, SKIING, SKATING, RUNNING, AND TRIATHLONS STRETCHING ROUTINES

These movements are geared towards any activity that emphases lower body movements predominately.

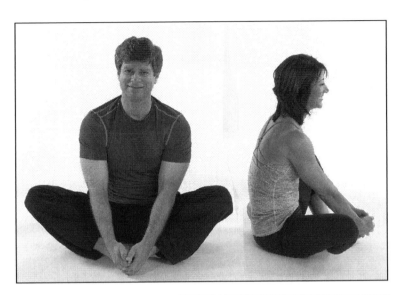

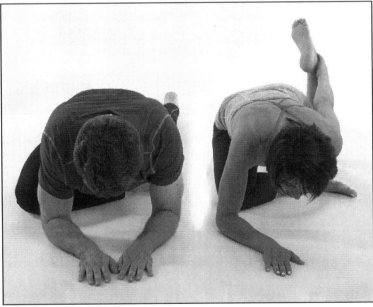

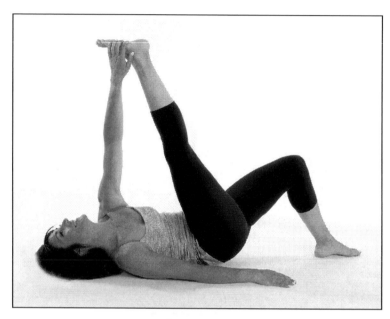

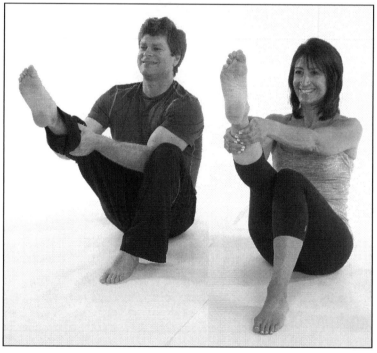

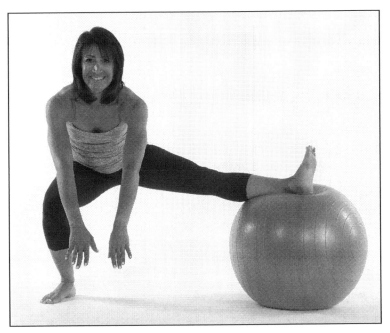

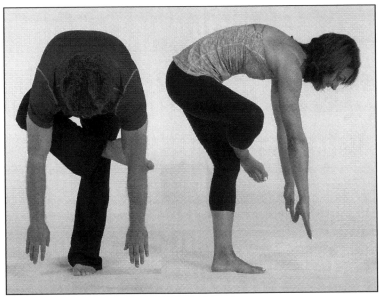

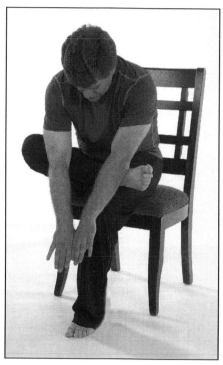

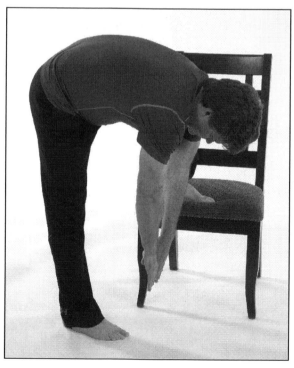

CLIMBING, MIX MARTIAL ARTS, KARATE, KICK BOXING, JUDO, WRESTLING, BOXING STRETCHING ROUTINES

These movements are geared towards any sport involving multi-tasking throughout the activity.

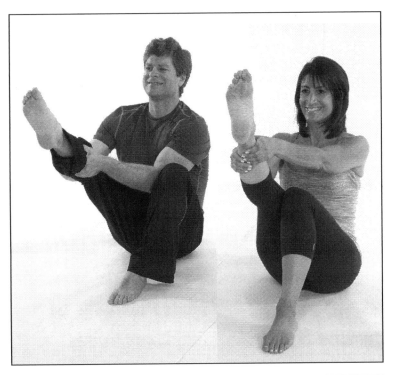

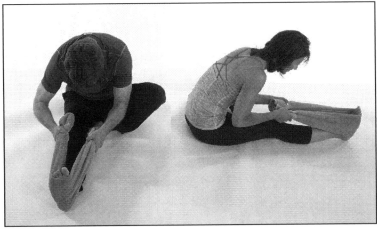

CLIMBING, MIX MARTIAL ARTS, KARATE, KICK BOXING, JUDO, WRESTLING, BOXING STRETCHING ROUTINES CONTINUED

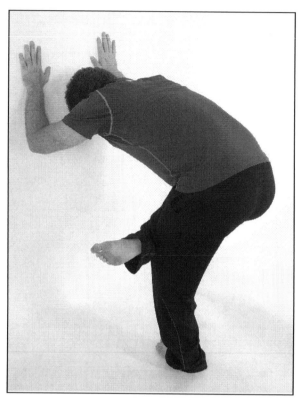

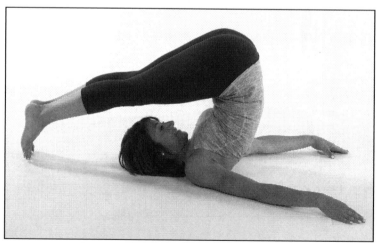

CLIMBING, MIX MARTIAL ARTS, KARATE, KICK BOXING, JUDO, WRESTLING, BOXING STRETCHING ROUTINES CONTINUED

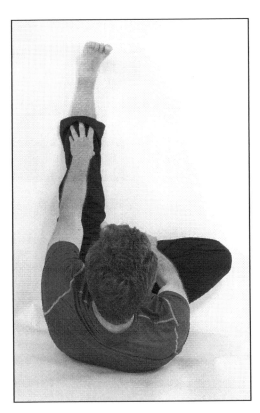

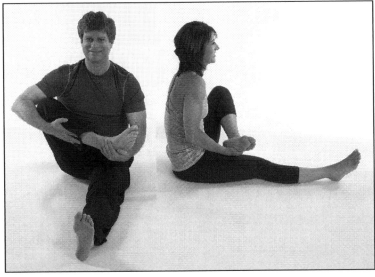

CLIMBING, MIX MARTIAL ARTS, KARATE, KICK BOXING, JUDO, WRESTLING, BOXING STRETCHING ROUTINES CONTINUED

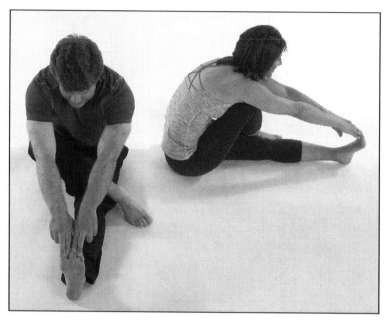

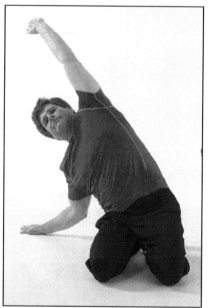

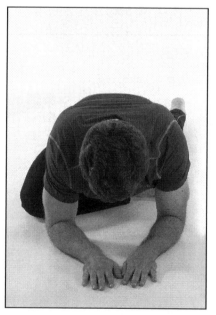

WALKING, HIKING, DANCING, JOGGING
STRETCHING ROUTINES

These movements are geared towards any sport involving steady pace activities.

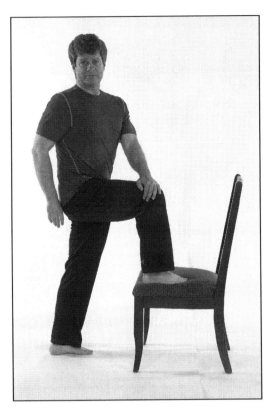

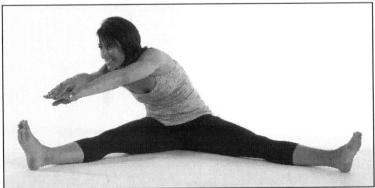

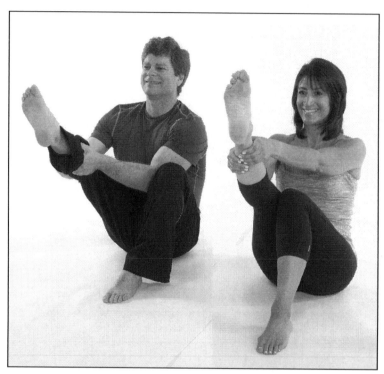

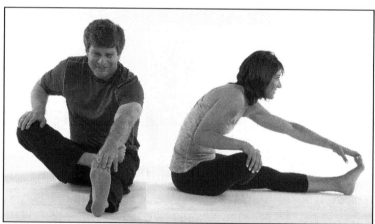

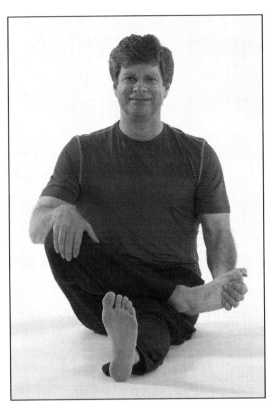

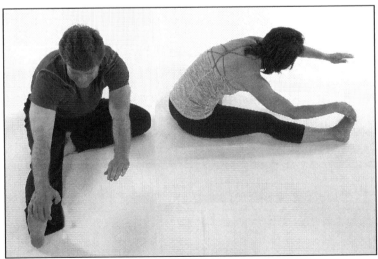

WALKING, HIKING, DANCING, JOGGING STRETCHING ROUTINES CONTINUED

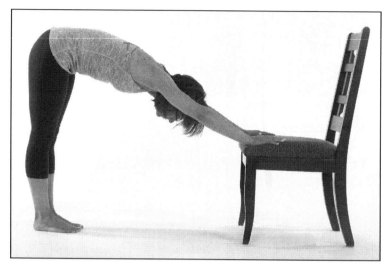

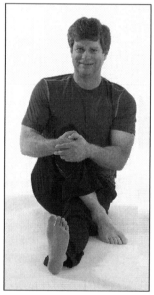

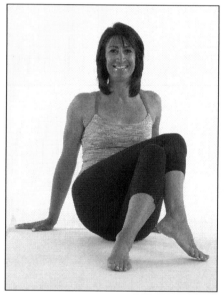

DESK JOCKEY, COMPUTER USER, AIR TRAVELERS STRETCHING ROUTINES

These movements are geared towards anyone in static positions long periods at a time.

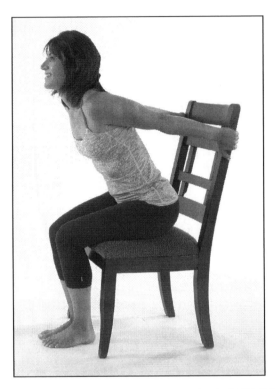

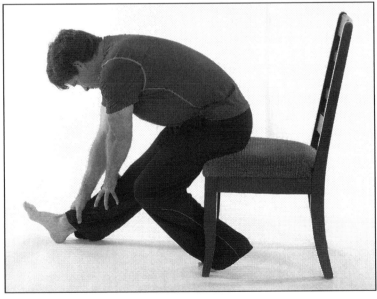

DESK JOCKEY, COMPUTER USER, AIR TRAVELERS
STRETCHING ROUTINES CONTINUED

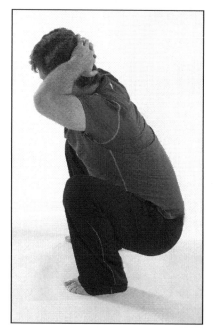 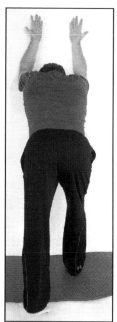

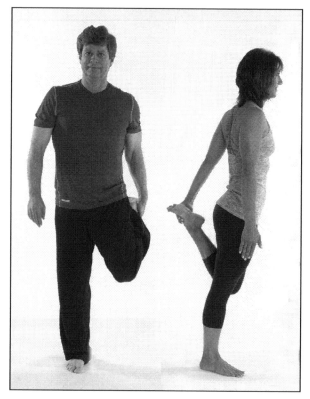

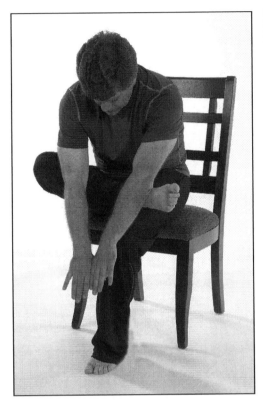

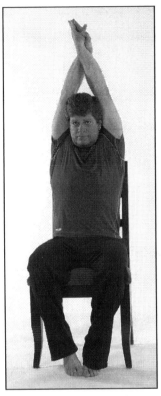

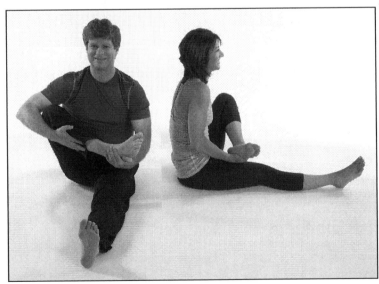

**DESK JOCKEY, COMPUTER USER, AIR TRAVELERS
STRETCHING ROUTINES CONTINUED**

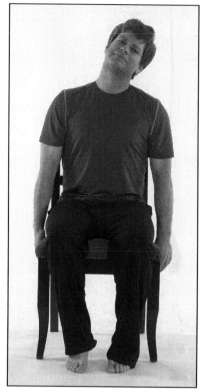 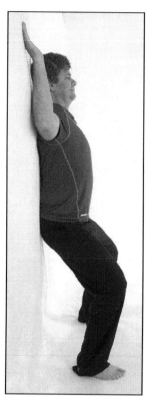

FULL BODY SHORT-ON-TIME STRETCHES
STRETCHING ROUTINES

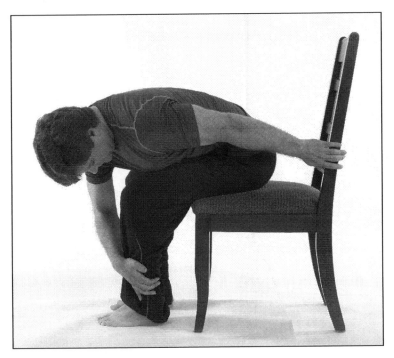

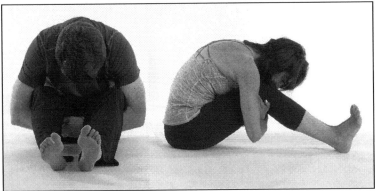

FULL BODY SHORT-ON-TIME STRETCHES STRETCHING ROUTINES CONTINUED

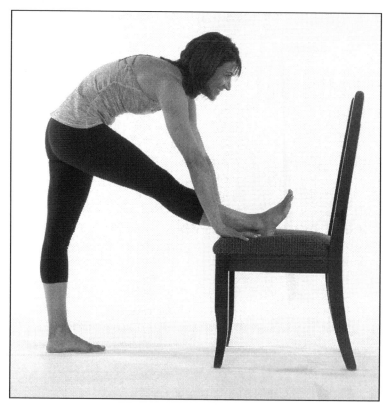

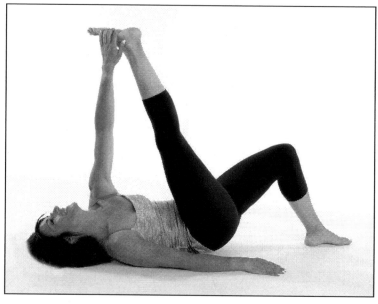

FULL BODY SHORT-ON-TIME STRETCHES STRETCHING ROUTINES CONTINUED

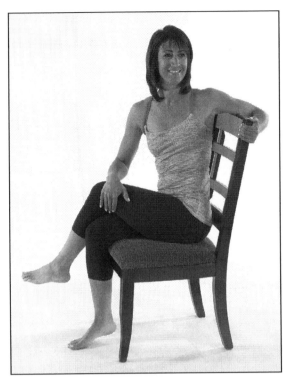

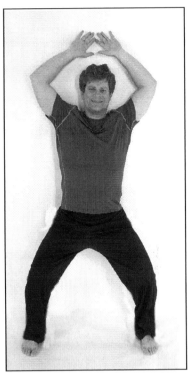

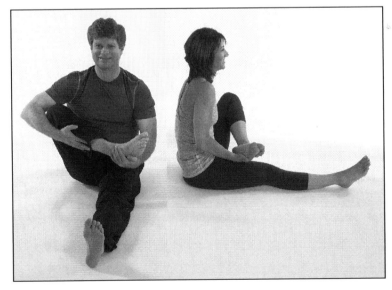

FULL BODY SHORT-ON-TIME STRETCHES STRETCHING ROUTINES CONTINUED

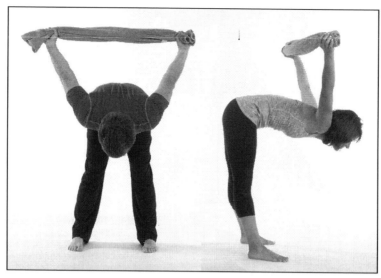

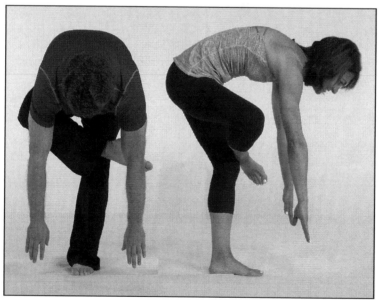

FINAL STRETCH

Release your tension. For the past two decades I have heard just about every excuses why someone is unable to achieve the flexibility they seek out. I hope after going through this book you can see this is untrue.

Restore—Follow the path of least resistance allowing yourself the easiest direction for your muscles to move in.

Re-balance—Focus on the action of the muscle groups as a whole rather than an individual muscle. This will help balance out your tight muscle groups with the more flexible area of your body.

Reconnect—Think of the *StretchSmart* movements as a repair manual. Use the stretches to relax your body gaining better control of your daily movements and sport related activities.

Patience—Let me take a moment to emphasize from the beginning of this journey. When you start a new exercise routine remember how sore you were the first few months of training? How about that first attempted mile rub out trying to hit a golf ball straight down the fairway? All of them needed practice and patience.

Now that you are armed with the *StretchSmart* system, I hope you will let it serve as a continual source of motivation and guidance, setting you on a course for a lifetime of greater flexibility and extraordinary fitness. As you can see, *StretchSmart* offers an enormous array of possibilities for stretching, allowing you to strive toward advanced levels of physical training. But remember, the challenge begins with you. Using all the guidelines that this book has to offer you, move intelligently, using one movement to guide you to the next advance range of motion.

I encourage you to pick up my two other books, *The BackSmart Fitness Plan* and *The Absmart Fitness Plan* for more stretches and exercise for a complete foundation of a training program. If you train right for your body type, eat well you will be able to perform at your optimal level each time you exercise.

Conversely, if you fail to challenge yourself or if you push too hard too quickly, you will undermine your efforts and become discouraged by doing the exercise halfheartedly will result in frustration. Listen to your body: push when you feel strong, go easy when you cannot give 100 percent, and adapt to your emotional as well as your physical well-being. If you do that, you will achieve your goals.

Each time you use a *StretchSmart* movement you are moving in the right direction. Wish you the best of health and success. Keep on training!

ABOUT THE AUTHOR

Adam Weiss is a board-certified chiropractic physician. Dr. Weiss graduated from National University of Health Sciences in 1992 and completed his clinical residency training at the Lombard and Chicago National Out-patient Centers. In addition, Dr. Weiss has completed more than 1800 hours of post-doctorate work in spinal rehabilitation, sport injuries and nutrition. Dr. Weiss has been in private practice for the past 24 years, specializing in neuromuscular injuries working with Olympic and professional athletes. A the medical director of PilatesSmart Fitness Center in Long Grove, Illinois, Dr. Weiss has been successfully integrating the *StretchSmart, AbSmart* and *BackSmart* methods, sports conditioning, and life-style changes including weight loss programs into his practice. Dr. Weiss's knowledge of flexibility, endurance, and strengthening exercise is a result of how own experience with martial arts and years of weight training and Pilates. He has held a first-degree black belt in Tae Kwon Do since the early age of 15, having competed in state and national competitions at the junior and senior levels.

Dr. Weiss is highly sought after as a team physician for Olympic and professional level athletes and young inspiring high school enthusiast. Dr. Weiss works with these athletes and teaches Pilates reformer cases daily while maintaining a full time practice. He also presents strengthening and conditioning exercise at workshops for professional and amateur sport clubs and martial arts studios throughout the United States.

Dr. Weiss own experience with back pain at an early age forced him to modify and adapt exercise routines, resulting in more productive and effective forms of exercise for people of all ages. Dr. Weiss has also written *The Backsmart Fitness* Plan: A total Body Workout to Strengthen and Heal Your Back, a complete fill body workout. *The AbsSmart Fitness Plan:* The proven workout to Lose Inches and Strengthen Your Core without Straining Your Back. Dr. Weiss has also contributed to national magazines on health and fitness based on these systems of toning and conditioning. Dr. Weiss has also been interviewed on Project Health Radio.

When not seeing patient, teaching Pilates, cooking, writing, reading and learning Japanese, he is experimenting with new exercises.

Previous books by Dr. Adam Weiss:

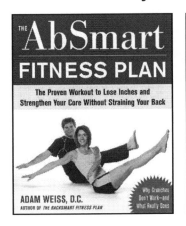 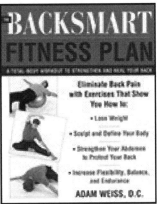

For more information regarding seminars, classes, DVDs, and future books

VISIT WWW.THEBACKSMART.COM

or search the internet with key words Dr. Adam Weiss, *AbSmart, BackSmart,* or *StretchSmart.*

To join *PilatesSmart* classes contact
Dr. Adam Weiss at
847-541-8844
in downtown Long Grove, Illinois

Made in the USA
San Bernardino, CA
09 December 2018